High-Yield Psychiatry
2nd edition

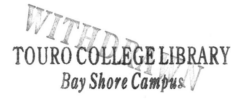
High-Yield Psychiatry
2nd edition

Barbara Fadem, Ph.D.

Professor of Psychiatry

Department of Psychiatry

University of Medicine and Dentistry of New Jersey

New Jersey Medical School

Newark, New Jersey

Steven S. Simring, M.D., M.P.H.

Associate Professor of Psychiatry

Vice Chair for Education and Training

Department of Psychiatry

University of Medicine and Dentistry of New Jersey

New Jersey Medical School

Newark, New Jersey

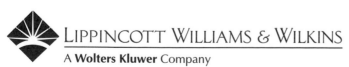

LIPPINCOTT WILLIAMS & WILKINS

A **Wolters Kluwer** Company

Philadelphia • Baltimore • New York • London
Buenos Aires • Hong Kong • Sydney • Tokyo

Editor: Neil Marquardt
Managing Editor: Beth Goldner
Marketing Manager: Scott Lavine
Production Editor: Jennifer D. Weir
Designer: Risa Clow
Compositor: Peirce Graphic Services
Printer: Data Reproductions Corporation

Printed in the United States of America

First Edition, 1998

Library of Congress Cataloging-in-Publication Data

Fadem, Barbara.
  High-yield psychiatry / Barbara Fadem, Steven S. Simring.—2nd ed.
    p. ; cm.
  Includes bibliographical references and index.
  ISBN 0-7817-4268-4
    1. Psychiatry—Outlines, syllabi, etc. 2. Mental illness—Outlines, syllabi, etc. 3. Psychotherapy—Outlines, syllabi, etc. I. Simring, Steven S. II. Title.
  [DNLM: 1. Mental Disorders—Outlines. 2. Psychotherapy—Outlines. WM 18.2 F144hf 2003]
  RC457.2.F343 2003
  616.89—dc21

                          2002043273

To purchase additional copies of this book, call our customer service department at **(800) 638-3030** or fax orders to **(301) 824-7390.** International customers should call **(301) 714-2324.**

Visit Lippincott Williams & Wilkins on the Internet: http://www.LWW.com. Lippincott Williams & Wilkins customer service representatives are available from 8:30 am to 6:00 pm, EST.

03 04 05 06 07
1 2 3 4 5 6 7 8 9 10

Contents

Preface

High-Yield Psychiatry, second edition, is designed to provide medical students with a clear, succinct presentation of topics seen on USMLE Step 2. Because many Step 2 questions require students to identify specific clinical syndromes from brief descriptions, we developed the concept of the "patient snapshot"—designated by the icon ⚫ —to provide memorable clinical portraits of psychiatric disorders.

Information about psychiatry is important in many aspects of medical education. In addition to material on clinical syndromes, this book includes special chapters on psychological issues in medical illness, medication-induced psychiatric symptoms, child and elder abuse, and ethics and legal medicine. Because of the limited time available to medical students, the information contained in all 30 of these chapters is presented in concise outline text form and in many quick-access tables. Each chapter and table provides a relevant "bite" of information for the mastery of the important USMLE Step 2 milestone in medical education.

Acknowledgments

We warmly thank Beth Goldner and the staff of Lippincott Williams & Wilkins for their assistance with the manuscript for this second edition. We are grateful also to the reviewers for their helpful suggestions and positive comments. We also acknowledge with great affection our loving, supportive spouses (Sue and Tom), children (Daniel, Eric, Jennifer, Jonathan, Kira, and Owen), and grandchildren (Joseph and Sarah). Finally, and as always, we are deeply in debt to the bright, hard-working medical students who have responded so enthusiastically to our efforts.

1

Classification of Psychiatric Disorders

I. THE *DIAGNOSTIC AND STATISTICAL MANUAL OF MENTAL DISORDERS, 4TH EDITION-TEXT REVISION*

A. The multiaxial system

    1. The *Diagnostic and Statistical Manual of Mental Disorders,* 4th edition (DSM-IV), published by the American Psychiatric Association, codes diagnoses of specific psychiatric illnesses along a multiaxial system.

    2. The DSM-IV-TR (text revision) is the latest version and contains a number of text changes which are included in this book.

    3. For each illness, the history and clinical presentation of the patient are matched with specific diagnostic criteria.

    4. The patient's condition is then coded along **five axes.** A definitive diagnosis can be made using only the first three axes (Table 1-1).

B. Subtypes and specifiers

    1. According to the DSM-IV classification, psychiatric disorders are divided into **subtypes** depending on the **presentation of symptoms** (e.g., schizophrenia, paranoid type).

    2. Illnesses also have **specifiers** that:

        a. Denote the **specific features** of an illness (e.g., major depressive disorder with psychotic features)

        b. Define the **severity** of the illness (e.g., mild, moderate, severe)

        c. Describe whether the illness is in **partial or full remission**

        d. Disclose the patient's **history** of the disorder

        e. Can be **provisional** if the practitioner believes that the full criteria for the disorder will be met over time

        f. Can include **"not otherwise specified"** (NOS) if the illness is atypical or does not clearly meet the criteria for a specific disorder because:

            (1) The disorder causes obvious distress, but is not listed in the DSM-IV-TR

            (2) The disorder meets some of the criteria for one or more conditions

            (3) An organic condition may be responsible for the symptoms

            (4) Not enough information is available to permit full classification

II. PSYCHIATRIC DIAGNOSTIC CRITERIA

A. **Major DSM-IV-TR diagnostic groupings.** The DSM-IV-TR includes 16 major diagnostic groupings, plus a grouping called "other conditions that may be a focus of clinical attention" (Table 1-2).

Table 1-1.

Axes of the *Diagnostic and Statistical Manual of Mental Disorders*, 4th Edition-Text Revision

Axis	Definition	Examples or Description
I	Clinical disorders	Major depressive disorder, schizophrenia
	Other disorders that may be a focus of clinical attention	Medication-induced disorder, malingering
II	Personality disorders	Personality characteristics that may be overshadowed by the Axis I diagnosis, but are long-standing and enduring and often have a profound effect on patient functioning
	Mental retardation	Intelligence quotient (IQ) < 70
III	General medical conditions	Physical illnesses that may be related to or affect a psychiatric problem
IV	Psychosocial and environmental problems	Divorce, death of a spouse, loss of a job
V	Global assessment of functioning (GAF)	Quantification of the patient's overall level of functioning in daily life using the GAF Scale (range, 1–100, from danger to oneself or others to superior functioning)

B. Practical psychiatric classifications

   1. Psychotic illnesses

      a. **Psychosis** is characterized by **loss of touch with reality** that causes problems in daily functioning.

      b. Psychotic symptoms include **hallucinations and delusions.**

      c. Psychotic symptoms are seen in illnesses such as schizophrenia, major mood disorders (e.g., bipolar disorder), and cognitive disorders (e.g., delirium).

   2. "Neurotic" illnesses

      a. Although the term "neurosis" is no longer used in diagnoses, the word is useful to describe a heterogeneous group of illnesses characterized by **problems functioning** in daily life and significant personal distress, but **no break with reality.**

      b. Neurotic symptoms include anxiety, excessive worrying, obsessions, and compulsions.

      c. Neurotic symptoms are seen in illnesses such as mood disorders, somatoform disorders, and anxiety disorders.

   3. Organic mental disorders

      a. The term **"organic mental disorders"** is no longer used because of the theoretical difficulty involved in separating organic from nonorganic disorders, because all psychiatric symptoms are mediated by the brain.

      b. The term "organic" is still useful, however, to suggest gross **anatomic abnormality** or **metabolic derangement** with cognitive impairment.

      c. An organic cause of psychiatric symptoms is likely if the patient:

         (1) Is disoriented or confused

         (2) Has a significant medical illness

         (3) Has a history of drug abuse

         (4) Has a sudden onset of symptoms

         (5) Has no family or personal history of psychiatric illness

   4. **Personality disorders** (coded on Axis II; see Chapter 21)

Table 1-2.
Organization of the *Diagnostic and Statistical Manual of Mental Disorders*, 4th Edition-TR

Category	Examples
Disorders usually first diagnosed in infancy, childhood, or adolescence	Mental retardation, learning disorders, motor skills disorder, communication disorders, attention-deficit and disruptive behavior disorders
Delirium, dementia, and amnestic and other cognitive disorders (formerly called "organic mental disorders")	Delirium due to congestive heart failure, dementia of the Alzheimer type
Mental disorders due to a general medical condition (formerly called "psycho-physiological disorders")	Catatonic disorder or personality change due to toxemia
Substance-related disorders	Alcohol-related disorders, amphetamine abuse, cannabis-induced disorders
Schizophrenia and other psychotic disorders	Schizophrenia, schizophreniform disorder, brief psychotic disorder
Mood disorders	Major depressive disorder, bipolar disorder
Anxiety disorders	Panic disorder, social phobia, posttraumatic stress disorder
Somatoform disorders	Somatization disorder, conversion disorder, hypochondriasis
Factitious disorders	Factitious disorder with predominantly psychological signs and symptoms or with predominantly physical signs and symptoms
Dissociative disorders	Dissociative amnesia, dissociative fugue, dissociative identity disorder
Sexual and gender identity disorders	Sexual dysfunctions, paraphilias, gender identity disorders
Eating disorders	Anorexia nervosa, bulimia nervosa
Sleep disorders	Primary sleep disorders, sleep disorders related to another mental disorder
Impulse-control disorders not elsewhere classified	Intermittent explosive disorder, kleptomania, pyromania, pathological gambling
Adjustment disorders	Adjustment disorder with depressed mood, adjustment disorder with anxiety, adjustment disorder with disturbance of conduct
Personality disorders	Paranoid personality disorder, schizoid personality disorder, antisocial personality disorder
Other conditions that may be a focus of clinical attention	Medication-induced movement disorders, relational problems, problems related to abuse or neglect, malingering
Additional codes	Unspecified mental disorder (nonpsychotic), no diagnosis or condition on Axis I

    a. Personality disorders are conditions that are characterized by **pervasive problems in social adjustment** or in **interpersonal relationships.**

    b. A patient with a personality disorder usually **does not directly experience distress;** however, his relatives, friends, and coworkers are affected negatively by his behavior.

    c. The patient may be upset over the consequences of a personality disorder, but usually has **no insight** into the fact that his behavior is the cause.

2

The Clinical Interview and the
Mental Status Examination

I. THE CLINICAL INTERVIEW

A. Function

    1. To establish **rapport** with and trust in the patient

    2. To elicit physical, psychological, and social **information** to help identify the patient's problem

    3. To obtain the patient's **psychiatric history,** including information about mental illnesses, drug and alcohol use, sexual activity, current living situation, and sources of stress

B. Table 2-1 shows examples of interviewing techniques.

II. THE MENTAL STATUS EXAMINATION

A. The mental status examination (MSE) is a **comprehensive survey of the current state of the patient's mental functioning.**

B. The MSE assesses a variety of characteristics, including general presentation (i.e., appearance, behavior, attitude toward the examiner), sensorium and cognition (i.e., level of consciousness, orientation, memory, attention, concentration, cognitive ability, spatial ability, abstraction ability), speech, mood and affect, thought (process and content), perceptual abilities, judgment and insight, reliability, and impulse control (Table 2-2).

C. The Folstein Mini-Mental State Examination (MMSE) is a commonly used bedside test that estimates cognitive impairment and tracks improvement or deterioration (Table 2-3). Batteries of psychological or neuropsychological tests are used for more comprehensive assessment of cognitive functioning (see Chapter 3).

Table 2-1.
Interviewing Techniques

Technique	Specific Function	Example
	TO ESTABLISH RAPPORT	
Support	To express the physician's interest in and concern for the patient	"That must have been a frightening experience for you."
Empathy	To express the physician's personal understanding of the patient's problem	"I can see that you're worried about the financial consequences of this injury."
Validation	To give credence and value to the patient's feelings	"Many people would also feel angry if they had been injured as you were."
	TO GATHER INFORMATION	
Open-ended question	To obtain as much information as possible without leading the patient and without closing off potential areas of pertinent information	"Tell me about your fear."
Facilitation	To encourage the patient to elaborate on an answer; may be a verbal question or body language (e.g., a quizzical expression)	"And then what happened?"
Reflection	To encourage the patient to expand on the answer by repeating part of the patient's previous response	"You said that your pain increased after you bent down to pick up the toy?"
Silence	To increase the patient's responsiveness	Waiting silently for the patient to speak
	TO CLARIFY INFORMATION	
Direct question	To elicit information from the patient quickly in an emergency situation; typically requires only a "yes" or "no" answer	"Have you taken penicillin before?"
Confrontation	To point out inconsistencies in the patient's responses or body language	"You say that you're not worried about tomorrow's surgery, but you seem nervous to me."
Recapitulation	To summarize the information obtained during the interview to ensure that the clinician understands it	"Let's go over what happened last night. You fell and hurt your side. Then you called the emergency squad, and they took you to the hospital, where you were examined in the emergency room."

Table 2-2.
The Mental Status Examination

Category	Characteristic	Example
General presentation	Appearance: Posture Grooming Appearance for age Clothing	 Has a hunched posture while standing Is unshaven Appears younger than his chronological age Is dressed inappropriately for the situation
	Behavior: Mannerisms Psychomotor behavior Tics	 Shows unusual facial expressions or hand movements Uses unusually quick (agitated) or slow (retarded) movements Uses repetitive, nonproductive movements
	Attitude toward the examiner: Reliable Cooperative Seductive Hostile Defensive	 Provides apparently correct historical information Follows the interviewer's instructions Behaves provocatively Seems angry Seems to take remarks personally
Sensorium and cognition	Level of consciousness: Lethargy Sleepiness	Has a Glasgow Coma Scale score of 3 (comatose) to 15 (completely alert) Seems mentally slowed down Seems tired
	Orientation: Person Place Time	 Does not know her name or with whom she lives Does not know where she is Does not know the year, day, or time
	Memory: Immediate Recent Remote	 Cannot remember three words when questioned after 5 minutes Cannot remember her activities during the last 12 hours [verify information to exclude confabulation (filling in memory gaps with false information)] Cannot remember basic historical information about herself (e.g., her city of birth)
	Attention Concentration Cognitive ability Spatial ability Abstraction ability	Cannot pay attention without being distracted by other stimuli Cannot repeat a string of three to six numbers forward and backward (digit span) or spell the word "world" backward Cannot read a simple paragraph of text. Does not know how many states make up the United States. Cannot compute 8×6 Cannot copy a simple drawing of a triangle or a square Cannot describe how a pear and an apple are alike Cannot explain the meaning of the proverb: "People who live in glass houses should not throw stones"

(continued)

Table 2-2.—*Continued*
The Mental Status Examination

Category	Characteristic	Example
Speech	Volume	Speaks too softly
	Speed	Seems compelled to speak quickly (pressured speech)
	Articulation	Does not speak clearly
	Deficiencies in language	Uses words incorrectly or has a poor vocabulary
Mood and affect	Mood	Describes feeling depressed (e.g., low, hopeless, suicidal) or manic (e.g., high, euphoric, irritable)
	Affect	Demonstrates to the examiner decreased (i.e., blunted, restricted, flat) external expression of mood
	Congruence and appropriateness	Described mood is similar to visible affect; both are appropriate to the situation
Thought	Form or process of thought (associations between thoughts)	Has thought patterns that make sense and follow each other logically
		Has thoughts that move rapidly from one to the other (flight of ideas)
		Repeats thoughts over and over (perseveration)
		Responds to the sound rather than the meaning of a word (echolalia)
	Content of thought:	
	Compulsion	Cannot refrain from performing an act (e.g., washing his hands)
	Obsession	Cannot get an unwanted thought out of his head
	Phobia	Has irrational fear (e.g., afraid to urinate in a public restroom)
	Delusion	Has false belief (e.g., is convinced that the CIA is after her)
	Idea of reference	Believes that an actor in a movie is talking about her
Perception	Illusion	Misinterprets reality (e.g., thinks that a toy on the floor in a dark room is a live snake)
	Hallucination	Has false sensory perception (e.g., sees a snake when there is nothing there)
Self-awareness	Judgment	Provides an unusual response to a hypothetical situation (e.g., says that he would discard a stamped, addressed letter that he found on the sidewalk)
	Insight	Understands that her symptoms are a result of her illness
Impulse control	Aggressive and sexual impulses	Cannot control impulses (based on the history and current behavior)

Table 2-3.
Folstein Mini-Mental State Examination*

Category	Sample Instructions to the Patient	Maximum Score
Orientation	Name the current location, time	10
Registration	Repeat the names of three objects	3
Attention and calculation	Subtract 7 from 100 and continue subtracting 7s	5
Recall	Recall the names of the above three objects	3
Language	Name the object I am holding	8
Construction	Copy this design	1

*Maximum total score = 30; total score <25 suggests some cognitive problems; total score <20 means definite impairment.

3

Diagnostic Tests

I. OVERVIEW

A. Types of tests

1. Psychological tests assess cognitive functioning (including intelligence), achievement, personality, and psychopathology.

2. The tests are classified by their purpose and by whether information is gathered objectively or projectively.

B. Objective versus projective tests

1. An **objective test** is based on questions with right or wrong answers that are **easily scored** and statistically analyzed.

2. A **projective test** requires the subject and the examiner to **interpret the questions. Responses** are assumed to be based on the subject's motivational state and defense mechanisms.

II. COGNITIVE TESTS

A. Intelligence and mental age

1. Intelligence is defined as the ability to understand abstract concepts; to reason; to assimilate, recall, analyze, and organize information; and to meet the special needs of new situations.

2. Mental age (MA), as defined by Alfred Binet, is a person's level of intellectual functioning.

B. Intelligence quotient (IQ)

1. On the Stanford-Binet and Wechsler Intelligence Scales (Table 3-1), IQ is the ratio of MA to chronological age (CA) multiplied by 100:

$$MA/CA \times 100$$

2. An **IQ of 100** means that the MA and CA are the same.

3. IQ is **relatively stable throughout life.** The highest CA used to determine IQ is 15 years.

4. The results of IQ tests are **influenced by culture and early experiences.**

5. Normal, or average, IQ is 90–109. The standard deviation in IQ scores is 15 points.

6. About fifty percent of the population falls in the average range.

Table 3-1.
Psychological and Neuropsychological Diagnostic Tests Used in Psychiatry

Category of Test	Test	Uses and Characteristics
Intelligence	Wechsler Adult Intelligence Scale—revised (WAIS-R)	Most commonly used intelligence test; 11 subtests (6 verbal and 5 performance) that evaluate general information, comprehension, similarities, arithmetic, vocabulary, picture assembly, picture completion, block design, object assembly, digit span, and digit symbol
	Wechsler Intelligence Scale for Children—revised (WISC-R)	Used to test intelligence in children 6–16½ years of age
	Wechsler Preschool and Primary Scale of Intelligence (WPPSI)	Used to test intelligence in children 4–6½ years of age
Achievement	Wide-Range Achievement Test (WRAT)	Used clinically to evaluate arithmetic, reading, and spelling skills
	Peabody Individual Achievement Test	Used in school systems to evaluate achievement in specific subject areas
Personality (used to identify personality characteristics and psychopathology)	Minnesota Multiphasic Personality Inventory (MMPI-2)	Objective test in which patients answer 567 true or false questions about themselves; clinical scales include depression, paranoia, schizophrenia, and hypochondriasis; validity scales measure "faking bad" (malingering) or "faking good" (hiding symptoms)
	Rorschach Test	Projective test in which patients interpret 10 bilaterally symmetric inkblot designs; used to identify thought disorders and defense mechanisms
	Sentence Completion Test (SCT)	Projective test in which patients complete sentences (e.g., I would most like to . . .); used to identify concerns and problems through verbal associations
	Thematic Apperception Test (TAT)	Projective test in which patients create scenarios based on 30 pictures of ambiguous situations; the scenarios are used to evaluate unconscious emotions and conflicts
Neuropsychological	Halstead-Reitan Battery (HRB)	Used to detect and localize brain lesions and determine their effects
	Luria-Nebraska Neuropsychological Battery (LNNB)	Used to determine left or right cerebral dominance and to identify specific types of brain dysfunction (e.g., dyslexia)
	Bender Visual-Motor Gestalt Test	Used to screen visual and motor ability through reproduction of designs

7. A score between 71 and 84 indicates borderline intellectual functioning.

8. A person with an IQ that is more than two standard deviations lower than the mean **(IQ < 70)** and meets other developmental criteria is considered **mentally retarded;** about 2.5% of the population falls in this range.

III. ACHIEVEMENT TESTS

A. Achievement tests evaluate how well an individual has mastered **specific subject areas.**

B. These tests are used in schools and industry (see Table 3-1).

IV. PERSONALITY TESTS AND MEASURES OF PSYCHOPATHOLOGY

A. Personality tests are used to evaluate **psychopathology and personality characteristics.**

B. The most commonly used personality tests [the Minnesota Multiphasic Personality Inventory (MMPI-2), the Rorschach Test, the Sentence Completion Test (SCT), and the Thematic Apperception Test (TAT)] are described in Table 3-1.

V. NEUROPSYCHOLOGICAL TESTS

A. Neuropsychological tests are designed to assess general intelligence, memory, reasoning, orientation, perceptuomotor performance, language function, attention, and concentration in patients with suspected neurologic problems (e.g., dementia, brain damage).

B. Specific neuropsychological tests are described in Table 3-1.

VI. BIOLOGIC EVALUATION OF THE PATIENT WITH PSYCHIATRIC SYMPTOMS

A. Measurement of biogenic amines and psychotropic drugs

1. Altered levels of catecholamines and their metabolites occur in some psychiatric conditions (Table 3-2).

2. Plasma levels of antipsychotic and antidepressant agents are measured to evaluate patient compliance and suspected overdose, and to determine whether therapeutic blood levels of the agent have been reached.

3. Levels of drugs of abuse are measured in body fluids **("tox screen")** to rule out substance-related causes of psychiatric symptoms (see Chapter 10).

B. Dexamethasone suppression test (DST)

1. In a normal patient with a normal hypothalamic-adrenal-pituitary axis, the synthetic glucocorticoid **dexamethasone suppresses the secretion of cortisol.** However, approximately one-half of patients with major depressive disorder have a positive DST (i.e., this suppression does not occur).

2. Positive DST findings are not specific. Nonsuppression is seen in conditions other than major depressive disorder, including schizophrenia, dementia, pregnancy, anorexia nervosa or severe weight loss, and endocrine disorders, and with the use, abuse, and withdrawal of alcohol and antianxiety agents.

C. Endocrine function

1. Thyroid function tests are used to screen for **hypothyroidism** and **hyperthyroidism,** which can **mimic mood disorders and anxiety.**

Table 3-2.
Biologic Evaluation of the Patient With Psychiatric Symptoms

Specific Test or Measure	Uses and Characteristics
NEUROENDOCRINE MEASURES	
Levels of biogenic amines (and their metabolites):	Measures levels of neurotransmitters and their metabolites in body fluids for diagnostic and research purposes
Dopamine (HVA)	Elevated in schizophrenia and other conditions involving psychosis; reduced in Parkinson disease and depression
Norepinephrine (VMA and MHPG)	VMA elevated in pheochromocytoma; MHPG decreased in severe depression
Serotonin (5-HIAA)	Decreased in severe depression, impulsiveness, violence, fire setting, Tourette syndrome, alcohol abuse, and bulimia
Dexamethasone suppression test (DST)	Used to predict which patients will respond well to treatment with antidepressant agents or to electroconvulsive therapy (i.e., those with a positive DST result, defined as reduced suppression of cortisol after test dose of dexamethasone)
Endocrine function	Used to identify hypothyroidism, which can cause symptoms of depression, or hyperthyroidism, which can cause symptoms of anxiety
NEUROIMAGING AND ELECTROENCEPHALOGRAM (EEG)	
Computed tomography (CT)	Identifies anatomic brain changes in cognitive disorders and possibly schizophrenia
Nuclear magnetic resonance imaging (MRI)	Helps to identify demyelinating disease (e.g., multiple sclerosis); shows the biochemical condition of neural tissues as well as the anatomy without exposing the patient to ionizing radiation
Positron emission tomography (PET), functional MRI (fMRI), or single photon emission computed tomography (SPECT)	Localizes areas of the brain that are physiologically active during specific tasks; characterizes and measures the metabolism of glucose in neural tissue
EEG and Q (quantitative) EEG	Measures (EEG) and quantifies (QEEG) electrical activity in the cortex; useful in diagnosing epilepsy and differentiating delirium (abnormal EEG) from dementia (often normal EEG)
Evoked EEG (evoked potentials)	Measures electrical activity in the cortex in response to touch, sound, or visual stimulation; used to evaluate vision and hearing loss in infants and brain responses in comatose patients and patients with demyelinating illness

(*continued*)

Table 3-2.—*Continued*

Biologic Evaluation of the Patient With Psychiatric Symptoms

Specific Test or Measure	Uses and Characteristics
OTHER TESTS	
Sodium amobarbital (Amytal; "truth serum") interview	Relaxes patients with conditions such as conversion disorder, mute psychotic states, and dissociative disorders so that they can express themselves during an interview
Intravenous administration of sodium lactate or inhalation of CO_2	Used to diagnose panic disorder because either treatment can provoke a panic attack in an affected patient
Galvanic skin response (part of the "lie detector" test)	Identifies level of stress as shown by arousal of the sympathetic nervous system; measures increased sweat gland activity that causes decreased electric resistance of the skin

HVA = homovanillic acid; VMA = vanillylmandelic acid; MHPG = 3-methoxy-4-hydroxyphenylglycol; 5-HIAA = 5-hydroxyindoleacetic acid.

2. Patients with **depression** may have **other endocrine irregularities** (e.g., reduced response to a challenge with thyrotropin-releasing hormone, abnormal regulation of growth hormone, reduced levels of melatonin and gonadotropin).

3. Psychiatric symptoms are also associated with other endocrine disorders, such as Cushing disease and Addison disease (see Chapter 22).

4. Other tests used to evaluate patients are shown in Table 3-2.

D. Laboratory tests to monitor patients for complications of pharmacotherapy

    1. Complete blood count (CBC) to screen for agranulocytosis in patients who are being treated with clozapine (Clozaril) or carbamazepine (Tegretol)

    2. Blood glucose test to screen for hypoglycemia, which can mimic depression, or hyperglycemia, which can lead to symptoms of delirium or anxiety

    3. Liver function tests in patients who are being treated with carbamazepine, valproic acid (Depakene), or divalproex sodium (Depakote)

    4. Thyroid function tests and renal panel in patients who are being treated with lithium

E. Neuroimaging and electroencephalogram (EEG) studies. Structural brain abnormalities and EEG changes may correspond to specific psychiatric disorders (see Table 3-2).

F. Other tests. Tests such as the sodium amobarbital interview, intravenous administration of sodium lactate or inhalation of CO_2, and galvanic skin response are used clinically, diagnostically, and for research purposes (Table 3-2).

4

Normal Child Development and Attention-Deficit and Disruptive Behavior Disorders

I. NORMAL CHILD DEVELOPMENT. Table 4-1 describes the motor, social, verbal, and cognitive characteristics of infants, toddlers, preschool children, school-age children, and adolescents.

   A. The infant (0–15 months)

   1. The **major psychological task** of infancy is to form an **intimate attachment to the mother or primary caregiver.**

   2. In a child between 6 and 12 months of age, **separation from the primary caregiver** results in initial protests and, if extended, by **anaclitic depression or "failure to thrive,"** also known as **reactive attachment disorder of infancy** (see Chapter 5).

   3. Failure to thrive is characterized by developmental retardation, poor health and growth, and a high death rate, despite adequate physical care.

   B. The toddler (15 months to 2½ years)

   1. The **major psychological task** of the toddler is to **separate from the mother or primary caregiver.**

   2. The child shows **"rapprochement,"** a tendency to move away from and then return to the mother for reassurance.

   3. When hospitalized, the toddler's greatest fear is separation from the mother, not physical injury or illness.

   4. The toddler can maintain a mental representation of an object even if it is no longer present **("object permanence").**

   C. The preschool child (2½ to 6 years)

   1. The child achieves **control over bowel and bladder** by 4 years of age and 5 years of age, respectively.

   2. Children in this age-group **do not understand the finality of death** and instead believe that dead people or pets will come back to life.

   3. Preschool children are very concerned about physical injury and illness **(the "Band-Aid" phase).** Thus, this age is a poor time to perform elective surgery.

   D. The school-age child (6–11 years)

   1. Psychosexual issues are relatively dormant during this period.

Table 4-1.

Motor, Social, and Verbal and Cognitive Development of the Normal Child

	Skill Area		
Age	**Motor**	**Social**	**Verbal and Cognitive**
2 to 3 months	Lifts head when lying on his stomach	Smiles in response to a human face ("social smile")	Coos, gurgles
5 to 6 months	Turns over, sits unassisted	Forms an attachment to primary caregiver, recognizes parents	Babbles (repeats a single sound over and over)
7 to 11 months	Crawls on hands and knees Pulls up to standing position	Shows fear in response to unfamiliar people ("stranger anxiety")	Imitates sounds, uses gestures
12 to 15 months	Walks unassisted	Fears separation from primary caregiver ("separation anxiety")	Says first words
16 months to 2½ years	Climbs stairs, scribbles on paper, uses a spoon, stacks 3–6 blocks	Plays independently, shows negativity (e.g., favorite word is "no")	Speaks in two-word sentences (e.g., "Me do."), names body parts and objects
2½ to 4 years	Rides a tricycle, undresses and partially dresses without help, copies a circle, line, or cross, identifies colors, stacks 9 blocks	Plays alongside, but not with, another child ("parallel play"), can spend much of the day with adults other than parents (e.g., preschool), develops core gender identity by 3 years of age	Speaks in complete sentences (e.g., "I can do it myself.") (beginning of Piaget's pre-operations stage)
4 to 6 years	Draws a person in detail (e.g., with arms, legs, body, eyes, hair); skips using alternate feet; buttons garments; ties shoelaces; copies a square or triangle; and rides a bicycle at 6 years of age	Plays cooperatively with other children; may have imaginary companions; has curiosity about the body, plays "doctor"; has romantic feeling about the opposite-sex parent (the "oedipal phase"); begins to develop moral values	Good verbal self-expression (e.g., tells detailed stories); begins to read at age 6 years
6 to 11 years	Engages in complex motor tasks (e.g., plays ball, rides a bicycle, skips rope)	Prefers to play with children of the same sex, is hardworking and industrious, develops a moral sense of right and wrong, learns to follow rules, identifies with the parent of the same sex, has relationships with adults other than her parents (e.g., teachers, group leaders)	Develops the capacity for logical thought; understands that objects have more than one property (e.g., can be both wood and blue); learns to read, write, and calculate (Piaget's "concrete operations" stage)

(continued)

Table 4-1.—*Continued*

Motor, Social, and Verbal and Cognitive Development of the Normal Child

Age	Skill Area		
	Motor	**Social**	**Verbal and Cognitive**
11 to 14 years	Has greater body strength, participates in individual and team sports	Shows preoccupation with gender roles, body image, and popularity; continues to separate from family; forms stronger relationships with peers	Develops abstract reasoning (beginning of Piaget's "formal operations" stage) and creativity
14 to 17 years	Shows motor skills that approach those of the adult	Has feelings of omnipotence that lead to risk-taking behavior (e.g., failing to use condoms, driving fast)	Continues development as intellectual capacity nears its peak
17 to 20 years	Reaches adult level of motor skills	Shows concern about humanitarian issues, morality, and self-control; may have an identity crisis that causes role confusion (manifested by criminal behavior or joining a cult)	Shows further development of abstract mathematic reasoning (e.g., calculus)

2. Children in this age-group **cope well with separation from their parents and tolerate hospitalization** reasonably well.

3. School-age children usually **comprehend the finality of death.**

E. The adolescent (11–20 years)

1. **In girls, puberty is defined as the first menstruation (menarche),** which occurs at approximately 11–14 years of age (much earlier than a century ago).

2. **In boys, puberty is defined as the first ejaculation,** which occurs at approximately 12–15 years of age.

3. Sexual drives are released through **masturbation,** which occurs in almost all adolescents.

4. Each adolescent wants to be like all other adolescents. For this reason, any alteration in expected developmental patterns (e.g., late menarche, acne, obesity) or chronic illness requiring changes in lifestyle (e.g., diabetes) may cause psychological distress.

II. ATTENTION-DEFICIT/HYPERACTIVITY DISORDER, CONDUCT DISORDER, AND OPPOSITIONAL DEFIANT DISORDER

A. General characteristics

1. These disorders are characterized by a child's **inappropriate behavior** that causes **difficulty in school performance and social relationships.**

2. **Frank mental retardation is not characteristic** of children with these disorders.

3. All of these disorders are **more common in boys.**

4. Examples ("patient snapshots"), patient characteristics, age of onset and occurrence, and prognosis of these disorders can be found in Table 4-2.

B. Differential diagnosis

1. Variants of normal temperamental characteristics and behavior

2. Mood disorders

3. Anxiety disorders

4. Specific learning disorders (e.g., dyslexia)

C. Etiology

1. **Genetic factors**

   a. There is a high concordance rate for attention-deficit/hyperactivity disorder (ADHD) in siblings.

   b. Relatives of children with conduct disorder and ADHD have an increased incidence of antisocial personality disorder and alcoholism.

2. Although there is no evidence of serious structural problems in the brain, **minor brain dysfunction** may be involved in the etiology of ADHD and conduct disorder.

3. Children with **conduct disorder** commonly have been **abused by caregivers.** The **parents** of these children often have a history of **substance abuse.**

4. In **oppositional defiant disorder,** there may be a history of **serious marital discord,** or **a mood disorder or substance abuse in one or both parents.**

D. Treatment

1. For **ADHD, central nervous system (CNS) stimulants** are the drugs of choice; **antidepressants** also may be helpful. CNS stimulants help lower activity level and increase attention span and ability to concentrate. These agents include:

   a. Methylphenidate [Ritalin; Concerta (extended release); $\leq$ 60 mg/day in children older than 6 years of age]

   b. Dextroamphetamine sulfate (Dexedrine; $\leq$ 40 mg/day in children older than 3 years of age)

   c. Amphetamine/dextroamphetamine [Adderall and Adderall XR (extended release); $\leq$ 30 mg/day in children older than 3 years of age]

2. **Adverse effects** of CNS stimulants in children include **failure to gain weight** and **inhibition of growth;** weight and rate of growth usually return to normal when the medication is discontinued

3. CNS stimulants may need to be taken for many years, sometimes beyond age 20, for "adult ADHD."

4. Children with conduct disorder and oppositional defiant disorder may benefit from a structured environment and psychotherapy, particularly family therapy (see Chapter 28).

Table 4-2.

Characteristics of Patients With Attention-Deficit/Hyperactivity Disorder, Conduct Disorder, and Oppositional Defiant Disorder

Disorder	Patient Snapshot	Characteristics	Age of Onset and Occurrence	Prognosis
Attention-deficit/hyperactivity disorder (ADHD)	An 8-year-old boy frequently gets into trouble at school because he interrupts the teacher, disturbs the other students, and cannot seem to sit still in class.	Overactivity; limited attention span; poor self-control; tendency to have accidents; impulsiveness; emotional lability; irritability; history of crying, high sensitivity to stimuli, and sleep problems in infancy	Onset before 7 years of age; lasting for at least 6 months; present in 3%–5% of children 5–12 years old; five times more common in boys; must occur in at least 2 settings (e.g., at home and in school)	20% of patients retain characteristics (e.g., limited attention span) into adulthood and remain at risk for mood and personality disorders; most children show complete remission during adolescence, with few long-term negative effects
Conduct disorder	An 8-year-old boy frequently gets into trouble at school because he hits the other children and has been found torturing the class guinea pig.	Behavior that violates social norms, including aggressive behavior toward others and toward animals, lying and stealing, destruction of property; serious deviation from societal and parental rules (e.g., truancy, setting fires)	Before 10 years of age for childhood-onset type; after 10 years of age for adolescent-onset type; occurs in 6%–16% of boys and 2%–9% of girls younger than 18 years of age	Associated with mood disorder, criminal behavior, antisocial personality disorder, and substance abuse in adulthood
Oppositional defiant disorder	An 8-year-old boy frequently gets into trouble at school because, although he gets along with the other children, he is belligerent toward the teachers and the principal.	A pattern of defiant, negative, noncompliant behavior toward authority figures, although this behavior does not grossly violate social norms; argumentative, angry, resentful, and easily annoyed	Onset before 8 years of age; occurs in 2–16% of children 6 to 18 years of age; onset before puberty is more common in boys; occurrence after puberty is equal in boys and girls	May progress to conduct disorder, remits in one-fourth of children

5
Childhood Mental Disorders

I. PERVASIVE DEVELOPMENTAL DISORDERS

A. Characteristics

    1. Pervasive developmental disorders are characterized by the **failure to acquire** or the **early loss of social skills and language,** resulting in lifelong problems in social and occupational functioning.

    2. These disorders include:

        a. Autistic disorder
        b. Asperger disorder
        c. Rett disorder
        d. Childhood disintegrative disorder

    3. These disorders are described in Table 5-1.

B. Differential diagnosis

    1. Congenital hearing impairment

    2. Psychosocial deprivation/neglect

    3. Schizophrenia with childhood onset

    4. Mixed receptive-expressive language disorder

    5. Obsessive-compulsive disorder

    6. Schizoid personality disorder

C. Etiology

    1. Perinatal complications

    2. Cerebral dysfunction

    3. Genetic component. The concordance rate for autism is at least 35% in monozygotic twins, lower in dizygotic twins. Some Rett cases are associated with an X-linked genetic abnormality.

D. Treatment

    1. There are no specific psychopharmacologic treatments.

    2. Behavioral therapy is used to increase social and communicative skills, decrease behavioral problems, and improve self-care skills.

    3. Because of the difficulties involved in caring for a child with a pervasive developmental disorder, **parents** usually benefit from **support and counseling.**

Table 5-1.
Pervasive Developmental Disorders of Childhood

Disorder	Patient Snapshot	Characteristics	Age of Onset and Occurrence	Prognosis
Autistic disorder	A 3-year-old boy shows no interest in or connection to his parents, other adults, or children. He does not speak voluntarily and is fascinated with watching rotating objects. He screams fiercely when his environment is altered in any way, such as when his mother tries to dress him	Severe problems in communication, but normal hearing; significant problems forming social relationships; repetitive behavior (e.g., spinning); self-destructive behavior (e.g., head banging); subnormal intelligence (IQ <70) in approximately two-thirds of patients; unusual specific abilities (e.g., exceptional musical ability) in some patients ("savant skills")	Onset before 3 years of age; seen in 0.02%–0.05% of children, although lesser forms are more common ("spectrum disorder"); three to five times more common in boys, but more severe when it occurs in girls	Most patients remain severely impaired in adulthood; only approximately 2% can work and live independently.
Asperger disorder	A 4-year-old boy has little interest in social interaction with his parents, other adults, or children and shows a variety of strange behavior patterns. His verbal and motor skills are appropriate for his age.	Significant problems forming social relationships; repetitive behavior; motor clumsiness; in contrast to autistic disorder, little or no developmental language delay and relatively normal cognitive development	First noticed at 3–5 years of age; incidence is unknown; more common in boys	Better prognosis than for autistic disorder

(continued)

Table 5-1.—*Continued*
Pervasive Developmental Disorders of Childhood

Disorder	Patient Snapshot	Characteristics	Age of Onset and Occurrence	Prognosis
Rett disorder	After 6 months of normal development, an infant begins to lose her acquired skills. By 18 months of age, she shows little social interaction with her parents, other adults, or children, and she uses strange hand gestures.	Diminished social interest and skills after a brief period of normal functioning; stereotyped hand-wringing movements; psychomotor abnormalities; mental retardation	Onset before 4 years of age (usually between 5 months and 48 months of age); seen only in girls; less common than autistic disorder	Progressive and lifelong, although social skills may improve somewhat with age
Childhood disintegrative disorder	A 4-year-old boy whose previous social and motor functioning was normal stops speaking and begins to crawl instead of walk.	Regression in verbal, motor, and social development after at least 2 years of normal functioning; mental retardation	Onset at 2–10 years of age; rare; may be more common in boys	Chronic and lifelong

II. TIC DISORDERS

   A. Tourette disorder

   1. Characteristics

   a. A 19-year-old man with normal intelligence and social relationships has had multiple motor tics since he was 8 years of age. At 17, he began to clear his throat intermittently and to utter strings of curse words during conversations.

   b. Tourette disorder is characterized by involuntary movements and vocalizations (tics).

   c. Patients often have many **motor tics** [e.g., facial grimacing, blinking (often the first tic seen), yawning].

   d. Most patients have at least **one vocal tic** (e.g., barking, grunting, involuntary use of profanity), which may appear years after the initial motor tics.

   2. Age of onset and occurrence

   a. The disorder **begins before 18 years of age,** usually with a motor tic that first occurs between 7 and 8 years of age.

   b. Tourette disorder occurs in approximately 0.05% of children.

   c. It is three times **more common in boys.**

3. Etiology

   a. Tourette disorder is associated with dysfunctional regulation of **dopamine** in the **caudate nucleus.**
   b. **Genetic factors**
       (1) The concordance rate is 50% in monozygotic twins and 8% in dizygotic twins.
       (2) Tourette disorder is genetically related to both attention-deficit/hyperactivity disorder **(ADHD) and obsessive-compulsive disorder.**

4. Treatment and prognosis

   a. Haloperidol (Haldol; 0.05–0.075 mg/kg/day) is the most effective treatment.
   b. Clonidine (Catapres) can improve tics.
   c. Pimozide (Orap; <10 mg/day) and the atypical antipsychotics like risperidone (Risperdal) are also effective.
   d. The disorder is **lifelong and chronic.**

B. **Chronic motor or vocal tic disorder** is characterized by involuntary motor tics or vocal tics, but not both. All other characteristics are similar to those of Tourette disorder.

III. ELIMINATION DISORDERS

A. Enuresis

   1. Characteristics and occurrence

       a. Enuresis is **voiding of urine** in inappropriate settings (e.g., in bed).
       b. Although most children are toilet trained during the daytime by 3 years of age, enuresis cannot be diagnosed before 5 years of age.
       c. It occurs in 7% of boys and 3% of girls at 5 years of age.

   2. Etiology

       a. Genetic factors (there is often a history of the condition in other family members)
       b. Physiologic factors, such as a small bladder and **naturally low nocturnal levels of antidiuretic hormone**
       c. Psychological factors, such as psychological stress caused by lifestyle changes (e.g., summer camp, moving, birth of a sibling)

   3. Treatment

       a. For nighttime enuresis, the **most effective treatment is behavioral** (e.g., a buzzer and pad apparatus, in which the buzzer sounds and wakes the child when the pad detects slight wetness).
       b. Pharmacologic treatments, including **imipramine** (Tofranil) and **antidiuretic compounds** such as intranasal desmopressin acetate (DDAVP), may be used in the short term for children who do not respond to behavioral methods.
       c. Support and reassurance for both the child and the parents are useful in combination with other treatments.

B. Encopresis

   1. Characteristics and occurrence

       a. Encopresis is soiling **(passage of feces)** in inappropriate settings.
       b. Most children are bowel trained by 3 years of age, but encopresis cannot be diagnosed in children who are younger than 4 years of age.

    c. It occurs in 1% of children at 5 years of age.

    d. It is three times **more common in boys.**

  2. Etiology

    a. Physiologic causes include **lack of sphincter control** and **constipation with overflow incontinence** (the most common form).

    b. Psychological causes include **regression** as a result of stress or power struggles with parents for autonomy.

  3. Treatment

    a. For physiological causes, laxatives and stool softeners to prevent constipation

    b. For psychological causes, psychotherapy, family therapy, and behavioral therapy

IV. OTHER DISORDERS OF CHILDHOOD

A. Selective mutism

  1. Characteristics

    a. *PATIENT SNAPSHOT* A 7-year-old girl does not speak in school, although she occasionally whispers to one friend. At home, she is appropriately talkative and social with family members.

    b. Typically, a child with this condition **speaks in some social situations** (e.g., at home), but not others (e.g., in school).

    c. The child may communicate nonverbally (e.g., with hand gestures).

    d. Selective mutism must be distinguished from normal shyness.

  2. Occurrence and etiology

    a. The condition is **rare,** occurring in fewer than 8 in 10,000 children.

    b. Selective mutism **occurs more frequently in girls.**

    c. The age of onset of this condition is commonly 5 or 6 years.

    d. The child often has experienced a **stressful life event** (e.g., moving, death of a loved one).

  3. Treatment and prognosis

    a. Family or behavioral therapy is the most effective treatment.

    b. Selective serotonin reuptake inhibitors (SSRIs) like fluoxetine (Prozac) may be helpful.

    c. Patients who remain mute after 10 years of age have a poorer prognosis.

B. Separation anxiety disorder

  1. Characteristics

    a. *PATIENT SNAPSHOT* Three months after moving to a new neighborhood, a 7-year-old boy refuses to sleep in his bed alone. He also refuses to go to school. When questioned about his behavior, he seems anxious and says that he is afraid that his mother will die.

    b. The child is very reluctant to be away from his parents because he has an **overwhelming fear of loss of his major attachment figures,** particularly his mother.

    c. This disorder has been called "school phobia." However, the child is actually fearful of leaving his parents, as opposed to being afraid of going to school.

    d. The parents are often overly concerned about the child.

    e. The child complains of physical symptoms (e.g., stomachaches or headaches) to avoid going to school and leaving the parents.

2. Occurrence and etiology

  a. It affects as many as 4% of grade-school children, with no sex difference.
  b. The most common age of onset is 7–8 years.
  c. The child often has experienced **a stressful life event** (e.g., moving, death of a loved one).
  d. Genetic or learning factors may be involved.
  e. **Anxiety disorders** are often present in the parents.

3. **Treatment and prognosis**

  a. **Family therapy** is effective.
  b. Treatment often involves gradual reintroduction to school and may include individual psychotherapy.
  c. **Antidepressants,** primarily imipramine (150–200 mg/day), are useful.
  d. Individuals with a history of separation anxiety disorder in childhood are at greater risk for anxiety disorders as adults, particularly **agoraphobia.**

C. **Reactive attachment disorder of infancy or early childhood**

  1. **Characteristics**

    a. _(PATIENT SNAPSHOT)_ A 22-month-old Russian boy who has been in an orphanage school since birth approaches and clings to every adult who enters the school playroom, even if he has never seen the person before.
    b. The child shows significant **disturbances in social relatedness.**
    c. There are two subtypes: the failure to respond in a socially normal way to others **(inhibited type)** and the formation of indiscriminate attachments to others **(disinhibited type).**
    d. The child may also show **developmental and physical delays** (i.e., "failure to thrive") (see Chapter 4).

  2. **Occurrence and etiology**

    a. Reactive attachment disorder is believed to result from severely pathological care, including neglect or abuse.
    b. It is more common in children exposed to repeated changes in environment and care-givers (e.g., in orphanages or foster homes).
    c. The condition is more common in single-parent and severely financially and socially stressed families.

  3. **Treatment and prognosis**

    a. Short-term hospitalization is used to protect the child and treat the malnutrition if present.
    b. Improving the family situation with interventions such as counseling, practical help with child care, and educating parents in child-care skills.

6

Aging, Geriatric Psychiatry, Death, and Bereavement

I. AGING

A. Demographics

   1. By the year 2020, more than 15% of the population of the United States will be 65 years of age or older.

   2. The overall average life expectancy of an American is about 76 years.

     a. Genetic factors are important determinants of life expectancy.

     b. Women live approximately 7 years longer than men.

     c. Because men are often some 2 years older than the women they marry, most married women will be widows for approximately 9 years.

     d. Although white Americans live longer than African Americans, this **difference between the races** (approximately 6 years in women and 8 years in men) is narrowing.

B. Physiological factors associated with aging

   1. Somatic factors

     a. Impaired vision, hearing, and immune response

     b. Decreased muscle mass and strength

     c. Increased fat deposits

     d. Osteoporosis

     e. Decreased gastrointestinal function

     f. Decreased renal and pulmonary function

     g. Loss of bladder control

     h. Decreased physiologic responsiveness to changes in ambient temperature

   2. Neural factors

     a. Decreased brain weight

     b. Enlarged ventricles and sulci

     c. Decreased cerebral blood flow

     d. **Senile plaques and neurofibrillary tangles** are present. These changes occur in the normally aging brain, but to a much lesser extent than in dementia of the Alzheimer type.

     e. **Minor forgetfulness.** In the normally aging person, slight problems with memory may be present, but they do not interfere with normal functioning (e.g., the patient may forget a doctor's appointment, but is well-groomed and lives independently).

   f. Absent brain disease, **intelligence quotient** (IQ) normally **remains stable** throughout life

  C. **Psychosocial factors associated with aging**

   1. Although some elderly people experience a sense of failure or despair about their lives, most are satisfied and proud of their accomplishments **("ego integrity").**

   2. Factors associated with **longevity**

    a. Marriage and other social support systems
    b. Advanced education
    c. Continued occupational and physical activity

II. PSYCHOPATHOLOGY IN THE ELDERLY

  A. **Depression**

   1. Depression is the **most common mental problem** in the elderly. **Suicide is twice as common in the elderly** as in the general population.

   2. Depression in the elderly is associated with the common losses of old age, such as:

    a. Deaths of family members and friends
    b. Decreased social status (e.g., retirement)
    c. Loss of health

   3. Because depression in the elderly is often associated with memory and cognitive problems, depression may be **misdiagnosed** as Alzheimer disorder **("pseudodementia").**

   4. Conversely, in its initial stages, loss of cognitive functioning in the elderly may present as depression or anxiety.

   5. **Treatment** for depression in the elderly includes supportive psychotherapy and **antidepressants,** particularly those with minimal anticholinergic activity, such as selective serotonin reuptake inhibitors (SSRIs) and secondary amine tricyclics. Electroconvulsive therapy (ECT) is also useful (Table 6-1; see also Chapters 13 and 25).

  B. **Other psychiatric problems**

   1. Certain other psychiatric disorders are more common in the elderly than in younger people because of anxiety-producing situations (e.g., physical illness) and the losses and stresses associated with old age.

   2. The cognitive disorders **delirium** and **dementia** (see Chapter 9) are also more common in the elderly.

   3. The **most common causes of delirium** in the elderly are

    a. **Physical illness** (e.g., myocardial infarction, cerebral infarction)
    b. **Vitamin or other nutritional deficiencies**
    c. The **effects of medications,** including side effects; adverse reactions; increased sensitivity to medications such as anticholinergic agents; drug interactions resulting from polypharmacy; and effects resulting from a decreased metabolic rate.

   4. These disorders and their treatment are described in Table 6-2.

III. DEATH AND BEREAVEMENT

  A. **Emotional responses to death or loss**

   1. When a patient is facing death or loss of a body part or function (e.g., mastectomy,

Table 6-1.
Treatment of Depression in the Elderly

Treatment	Comments	Dose or Schedule
Selective serotonin reuptake inhibitors (SSRIs)	Fewer life-threatening side effects (especially cardiovascular) than tricyclics	Start with a low dose (e.g., 10–20 mg/day fluoxetine or paroxetine; 25–50 mg/day sertraline) and increase gradually
Tricyclic antidepressants (TRCs)	Desipramine has relatively fewer anti-cholinergic effects; nortriptyline causes less orthostatic hypotension and has fewer cardiac effects	Start with a low dose (e.g., 10–25 mg/day) and increase gradually
Monoamine oxidase inhibitors (MAOIs)	Because many elderly people are hypertensive, there are additional concerns if a hypertensive crisis occurs after the ingestion of tyramine-containing foods; drug interactions may occur, particularly with analgesics [e.g., meperidine (Demerol)] and stimulants [e.g., dextroamphetamine (Dexedrine)]	Start with a low dose of phenelzine (e.g., 15 mg/day) and increase gradually. Pay careful attention to diet and drug–drug interactions
Electroconvulsive therapy (ECT)	Effective and possibly safer than antidepressants in the elderly	Give a course of eight treatments over 2–3 weeks; afterward, maintenance therapy ECT may be useful

diabetic retinopathy), she experiences five specific emotional changes, or stages (first described by Kübler-Ross).

2. These stages may occur in any order or simultaneously. Not every patient experiences all of the stages.

3. Stages of dying

    a. Denial. The patient refuses to believe that she has a terminal illness (e.g., "There is an error in the lab report.").

    b. Anger. The patient blames others for the illness (e.g., "The doctor should have had me come in more often.").

    c. Bargaining. The patient uses the defense mechanism of **undoing** (e.g., "I will never smoke again if the tumor goes away.").

    d. Depression. The patient becomes quiet, detached, and sad (e.g., "I feel like giving up right now.").

    e. Acceptance. The patient finally accepts her fate (e.g., "I have put my affairs in order and I am ready to go.").

B. Normal grief (bereavement) versus abnormal grief (depression)

    1. After a major loss (e.g., death of a loved one), a **normal grief reaction** can be expected to occur.

    2. After such a loss, normal grief or bereavement must be distinguished from abnormal grief or depression (e.g., major depressive episode, dysthymic disorder; Table 6-3).

Table 6-2.

Other Common Psychiatric Disorders in the Elderly and Their Treatment

Disorder (Chapter in *High Yield Psychiatry*)	Treatment
Insomnia (8)	Improved sleep hygiene; rapidly eliminated hypnotic benzodiazepines [e.g., temazepam (Restoril)] for short-term use only; nonbenzodiazepine sleep agents [e.g., zolpidem (Ambien)]
Adjustment disorders (20)	Short-term psychotherapy; drugs are rarely needed
Anxiety disorders (14)	Supportive psychotherapy, antidepressants and antianxiety agents, including: benzodiazepines (avoid long-acting agents that accumulate in adipose tissue); buspirone (start with 5 mg/day) causes less sedation and fewer problems with abuse, but full pharmacotherapeutic effect takes a few weeks; and antihistamines (e.g., diphenhydramine), which provide sedation with less potential for abuse than benzodiazepines but which may cause troublesome side effects in the elderly.
Alcohol-related disorders (often unidentified, but present in 10%–15% of the geriatric population (10)	Alcoholics Anonymous or another 12-step program; supportive psychotherapy; dietary supplements, especially B vitamins; rule out comorbid psychiatric illnesses ("dual diagnosis")
Hypochondriasis (15)	Evaluate for depression; regular visits to investigate objective signs of illness and to provide reassurance
Delusional disorder (12)	Antipsychotic agents (high-potency antipsychotics are less sedating; start with 1 mg/day haloperidol or 2 mg/day trifluoperazine); atypical antipsychotics like risperidone, psychotherapy
Delirium (9)	Resolution of the underlying medical or surgical problem
Dementia (with or without psychotic symptoms) (9)	Resolution of the underlying medical or surgical problem, when possible; structured environment; treatment of the associated symptoms (e.g., anxiety, depression); currently no effective long-term pharmacologic treatment for dementia of the Alzheimer type, although anticholinesterase agents, such as donepezil (Aricept 5–10 mg/day), may slow the progression of disease in some patients

Table 6-3.

Comparison Between Normal Grief (Bereavement) and Abnormal Grief (Depression)

Normal Grief	Abnormal Grief
A 68-year-old woman whose husband died 4 months ago appears well groomed and reports that although she often feels sad, she enjoys spending time with her children.	A 68-year-old woman whose husband died 4 months ago appears dirty and disheveled, has lost 12 pounds, and refuses to leave her house or to interact with friends and family.
Minor weight loss	Significant weight loss
Mild sleep disturbances	Significant sleep disturbances
Mild guilt	Strong feelings of guilt and worthlessness
Illusions (e.g., mistaking a live person for the deceased person)	Hallucinations (e.g., hearing the dead person talking) and delusions
Attempts to return to work and social activities	Resumes few, if any, social activities
Expresses sadness	Considers or attempts suicide
Severe symptoms resolve within 2 months	Severe symptoms persist for > 2 months
Moderate symptoms subside within 1 year	Moderate symptoms persist for > 1 year
Treatment includes increased calls and visits to the physician, supportive psychotherapy, and short-acting sedatives (but not barbiturates) for acute problems with sleep	Treatment includes antidepressants, antipsychotics, or electroconvulsive therapy

7

Child and Adult Abuse and Neglect

I. OVERVIEW OF CHILD ABUSE

A. Types of child abuse

    1. Sexual abuse

    2. Physical abuse (the "battered child syndrome")

    3. Emotional neglect (e.g., withholding of parental love and attention, rejection)

B. Occurrence and prognosis

    1. Reported child abuse is increasing, although most cases still are not reported.

    2. Adults who were abused as children are at greater risk for anxiety, depression, substance abuse disorders, dissociative disorders, posttraumatic stress disorder, and abusing their own children.

C. Role of the physician

    1. According to the law in every state, **physicians must report suspected physical or sexual abuse** of a child to the appropriate family social service agency.

    2. The physician also must **admit the child to the hospital** for protection when necessary and arrange for follow-up by social service agencies.

    3. The physician is not required to tell the parents that she suspects child abuse, and she does not need parental consent to hospitalize or treat the child.

II. SEXUAL ABUSE OF CHILDREN

A. Characteristics

    1. Most child sexual abusers are male.

    2. The child usually knows the abuser (e.g., father, stepfather, uncle, mother's boyfriend, family acquaintance); few are strangers to the child.

    3. Signs of sexual abuse in children are shown in Table 7-1.

B. Occurrence

    1. Child sexual abuse is now being reported more frequently than in the past; at least 250,000 cases are reported annually.

    2. Most sexually abused children are 9–12 years old, and 25% are younger than 8 years old.

    3. Approximately 25% of all girls and 12% of all boys report sexual abuse at some time during their lives.

Table 7-1.
Evidence of Abuse

	Patient Snapshot	Evidence of Abuse
Child sexual abuse	A 4-year-old girl tells the physician that her mother's boyfriend asked her to kiss his penis. Physical examination of the child is unremarkable.	• Specific knowledge about sexual acts (e.g., fellatio) in a young child • Genital or anal trauma • Sexually transmitted disease • Recurrent urinary tract infections • Excessive initiation of sexual activity with friends
Child physical abuse	A 5-month-old girl is brought to the emergency room unconscious. While no external injuries are seen, physical examination reveals a subdural hematoma, retinal hemorrhages, and retinal detachment (the "shaken baby syndrome" caused by shaking the child to halt its crying). The parents tell the physician that the child fell out of her crib.	• Neglect, such as poor personal care (e.g., diaper rash, dirty hair), lack of needed nutrition • Bruises, particularly in areas not likely to be injured during normal play, such as buttocks or lower back; internal abdominal injuries • Physical signs of restraint caused by tying to a bed or chair • Fractures at different stages of healing; spiral fractures caused by twisting the limbs • Cigarette burns • Burns on the feet or buttocks due to immersion in hot water • Belt marks
Elder abuse	A mildly demented 83-year-old man is brought to the emergency room by his daughter with whom he lives. He smells of urine, is undernourished, and has bruises on both of his arms. He denies that anyone has harmed him.	• Neglect such as poor personal care and hygiene, or lack of needed nutrition, medication, or health aids (e.g., eyeglasses, dentures) • Bruises; internal abdominal injuries • Physical signs of restraint caused by tying to a bed or chair • Fractures at different stages of healing; spiral fractures caused by twisting the limbs

C. Characteristics of the child abuser

1. Substance abuse

2. Marital problems and no appropriate alternate sexual partner

3. Immature, dependent personality

4. Occasionally, true pedophilia (preferential sexual desire for children; see Chapter 17)

III. PHYSICAL ABUSE OF CHILDREN

A. Characteristics

  1. Commonly, parents physically abuse only certain children (i.e., those perceived as slow, different, or difficult to control) and spare others.

  2. Characteristics of child physical abuse, including the **"shaken baby syndrome,"** are shown in Table 7-1.

B. Occurrence

  1. More than **1 million** substantiated new cases of child physical abuse and at least 2000–4000 abuse-related deaths occur annually.

  2. The most common abuser is the **mother.**

  3. Young children are the most likely to be abused: 33% of physically abused children are younger than 5 years of age, 25% are 5–9 years of age.

C. Characteristics of the abuser

  1. Personal history of victimization by caretaker or spouse

  2. Substance abuse

  3. Poverty

  4. Social isolation

D. Characteristics of the abused child

  1. Prematurity or low birth weight

  2. Hyperactivity or mild physical handicap

  3. Colicky or "fussy" as an infant

  4. Physical resemblance to the abuser's absent, rejecting, or abusive partner

IV. PHYSICAL ABUSE AND NEGLECT OF THE ELDERLY

A. Characteristics

  1. Many abused elderly people have some degree of **dementia** and are incontinent.

  2. The most likely abuser of an elderly person is the **spouse.** If the abused person is widowed, the daughter or son with whom he lives (and often supports financially) is the most likely abuser.

B. Occurrence. Approximately 1 million cases of elder abuse are reported annually; however, most cases are not reported.

C. The role of the physician in elder abuse

  1. Typically, the elderly person who is being abused does not report the abuse, but instead says that he fell and injured himself.

  2. Signs of elder abuse are shown in Table 7-1.

  3. When a physician suspects that an elderly person is being abused, she should **report the case** to the appropriate social service agency.

V. PHYSICAL AND SEXUAL ABUSE OF DOMESTIC PARTNERS

A. At least 2 million cases of domestic abuse occur annually. Many cases are not reported. The abuser is almost always male.

B. Physical evidence includes bruises (e.g., blackened eyes, bruises on the breasts) and broken bones.

C. The abused partner may not leave the abuser because:

1. She has nowhere to go.

2. He has threatened to kill her if she leaves. (In fact, she has a greatly increased risk of being killed by him at the time she leaves.)

D. The **cycle of abuse**

1. Buildup of tension in the abuser

2. Abusive behavior (battering)

3. Apologetic and loving behavior by the abuser toward the victim

E. A physician who suspects domestic abuse should provide emotional support to the abused partner, refer her to an appropriate shelter or program, and encourage her to report the case to law enforcement officials. Direct reporting by the physician (as in child abuse) is not appropriate because the victim is a competent adult, and it may put the victim at greater risk.

F. Characteristics of abusers and abused partners are shown in Table 7-2.

VI. SEXUAL ABUSE OF ADULTS: RAPE AND RELATED CRIMES

A. A 33-year-old woman who has a 4-year-old child comes to the emergency room and reports that she was raped by her boyfriend on a date 2 days ago. The examination shows no physical evidence of rape (i.e., no genital injuries, no semen). She appears anxious, disheveled, and "spacey."

B. Legal considerations

1. Rape is known legally as "sexual assault" or "aggravated sexual assault" and involves sexual contact without consent. Penetration by a finger, penis, or other object may or may not occur; erection and ejaculation do not have to occur.

2. Because rapists may use **condoms to avoid DNA identification or to avoid contracting human immunodeficiency virus (HIV),** or because they may have difficulty with erection or ejaculation, semen may not be present in the vagina of a rape victim.

3. Sodomy means oral or anal penetration. The victim may be male or female.

4. A victim is not required to prove that she resisted the rapist for him to be convicted. A rapist was convicted recently even though the victim begged him to use a condom.

Table 7-2.
Characteristics of Abusers and Abused Domestic Partners

Abuser	Abused Partner
Alcohol or drug abuse	Financial or emotional dependence on the abuser
Impulsivity and a low tolerance for frustration	Pregnancy (injuries are often on the breasts and
Displacement of angry feelings onto partner	abdomen, the "baby zone")
Low self-esteem	Dependency
	Self-blame
	Low self-esteem

5. Certain information about the victim (e.g., previous sexual activity, "provocative" clothing worn at the time of the attack) is generally not admissible as evidence in rape trials.

6. In almost every state, **husbands can be prosecuted** for raping their wives ("spousal rape"); it is illegal to force anyone to engage in sexual activity.

7. Consensual sex may be considered rape **("statutory rape")** if the victim is younger than 16 or 18 years old (depending on state law) or is physically or mentally handicapped.

8. Rape is a crime of violence, not of passion.

C. **Characteristics of the rapist**

1. Most rapists are **younger than 25 years of age.**

2. The rapist usually is the **same race as the victim and known to the victim.**

3. **Alcohol** use by the rapist occurs in at least one-third of rape cases.

D. **Characteristics of the victim**

1. The typical rape victim is between 16 and 24 years of age, although victims may be middle-aged or even elderly.

2. Rape most commonly occurs **inside the victim's home.**

3. Vaginal injuries may be absent, particularly in parous women.

E. **The aftermath of rape**

1. For a variety of reasons, including shame, fear of retaliation, and the difficulties in-

Table 7-3.
The Physician's Role in the Follow-up of a Rape Victim

Immediately after the Incident

- Take the patient's history (be supportive and nonjudgmental).
- Do not question the patient's veracity or judgment.
- Perform a general physical examination.
- Conduct laboratory tests (e.g., cultures for sexually transmitted diseases from the vagina, anus, and pharynx; test for presence of semen).
- Prescribe prophylactic antibiotics and postcoital contraceptive measures (e.g., mifepristone–RU486 [Mifeprex]) if appropriate.
- Encourage the patient to notify the police.

1–2 and 7 Days after the Incident

- Interview the patient and discuss emotional and physical sequelae of the rape (e.g., suicidal thoughts, vaginal bleeding).
- Do a pregnancy test.
- Allow the patient to express her anger.
- Refer the patient for counseling.
- Follow up on legal matters.

6 Weeks after the Incident

- Reevaluate the patient's physical status.
- Repeat tests for sexually transmitted diseases.
- Repeat laboratory test for pregnancy.
- Refer the patient for long-term counseling if appropriate.

volved in substantiating rape charges, **only 25% of all rapes are reported to the police.**

2. **Blaming the victim** is common in rape cases.

3. The length of the emotional recovery period after rape varies, but is commonly at least 1 year. **Posttraumatic stress disorder** sometimes occurs after rape (see Chapter 14).

4. The most effective type of counseling is group therapy with other rape victims.

5. The physician's role in the follow-up of rape cases is described in Table 7-3.

8

Normal Sleep and Sleep Disorders

I. NORMAL SLEEP

A. **Awake state.** Beta and alpha waves characterize the electroencephalogram (EEG) of the awake individual.

    1. **Beta waves** are seen with **active mental concentration.**

    2. **Alpha waves** are seen when a person **relaxes with eyes closed.**

B. **Sleep state.** During sleep, brain waves show distinctive changes (Table 8-1).

    1. Sleep is divided into REM (rapid eye movement) sleep and non-REM sleep, which consists of stages 1, 2, 3, and 4. Stages 3 and 4 together are called *delta*, or slow wave sleep.

    2. Sleep architecture maps the transition from one stage of sleep to another (Figure 8-1).

    3. During **REM sleep,** high levels of brain activity occur.

        a. Average time to the first REM period after falling asleep **(REM latency)** is 90 minutes.

        b. REM periods of 10–40 minutes each occur **about every 90 minutes** throughout the night.

        c. A person who is **deprived of REM sleep** one night (e.g., because of inadequate sleep or repeated awakenings) has increased REM sleep the next night **(REM rebound).**

        d. Prolonged REM deprivation or total sleep deprivation may also result in transient anxiety or psychotic symptoms.

C. Neurotransmitters involved in the production of sleep

    1. Increased levels of **dopamine** decrease total sleep time; treatment with antipsychotics, which block dopamine receptors, may improve sleep.

    2. Increased levels of **norepinephrine** decrease both total sleep time and REM sleep.

    3. Increased levels of **serotonin** increase both total sleep time and delta sleep. Damage to the dorsal raphe nuclei, which produce serotonin, decreases both of these measures.

    4. Increased levels of **acetylcholine** increase both total sleep time and REM sleep.

II. CAUSES OF SLEEP DISORDERS

A. Physical causes

    1. **Medical conditions** (i.e., pain, endocrine disorders)

Table 8-1.
Characteristics of Awake State and of Sleep Stages

Sleep Stage	Associated EEG Pattern	% Sleep Time in Young Adults	Characteristics
Awake	Beta Alpha	— —	Active mental concentration Relaxed with eyes closed
Stage 1	Theta	5%	Lightest stage of sleep characterized by peacefulness, slowed pulse and respiration, decreased blood pressure, and episodic body movements
Stage 2	Sleep spindle and K-complex	45%	Largest percentage of sleep time
Stages 3 and 4	Delta (slow-wave sleep)	25% (decreases with age)	Deepest, most relaxed stage of sleep; sleep disorders, such as night terrors, sleep-walking (somnambu-lism), and bed-wetting (enuresis) may occur
Rapid eye movement (REM) sleep	"Sawtooth," beta, alpha, and theta	25% (decreases with age)	Dreaming; penile and clitoral erection; increased cardiovascular activity; absence of skeletal muscle movement

Adapted from Fadem B: *BRS Behavioral Science,* 3e. Philadelphia, Lippincott Williams and Wilkins, 2000, p. 88.

2. **Withdrawal from drugs with sedating effects** (e.g., alcohol, benzodiazepines, phenothiazines, marijuana, opiates)

3. **Use of central nervous system (CNS) stimulants** (e.g., caffeine, amphetamines)

4. **Aging** is associated with repeated nighttime awakenings and reduced REM and delta (slow-wave) sleep.

B. **Psychological causes**

1. Patients with **major depressive disorder** have normal sleep onset, have repeated nighttime awakenings and **wake too early in the morning** (terminal insomnia). Short REM latency (REM occurs within a few minutes of falling asleep), long first

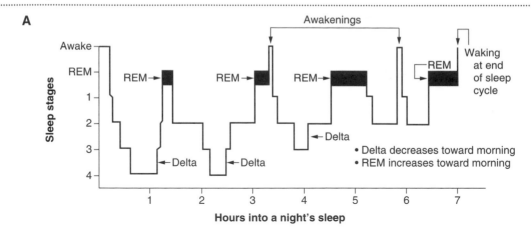

Figure 8–1. Sleep architecture in a normal young adult. REM = rapid eye movement. (Adapted from Wedding D: *Behavior and Medicine*. St. Louis, Mosby Year book, 1995, p. 416.)

REM period, increased REM early in the night and decreased REM later in the night, and reduced delta sleep may occur.

  2. Patients with **mania or hypomania** have trouble falling asleep and need little sleep.

  3. Patients with **anxiety disorders** often have trouble falling asleep.

III. CLASSIFICATION OF SLEEP DISORDERS. The *Diagnostic and Statistical Manual of Mental Disorders*, 4th edition (DSM-IV-TR), classifies sleep disorders into two major categories:

  A. Dyssomnias are characterized by problems in the timing, quality, or amount of sleep. They include insomnia, hypersomnia, narcolepsy, breathing-related sleep disorder (sleep apnea), and circadian rhythm sleep disorder.

  B. Parasomnias are characterized by abnormalities in physiology or in behavior associated with sleep. They include sleepwalking, sleep terror disorder, and nightmare disorders.

  C. Insomnia, narcolepsy, and breathing-related sleep disorder are described below and in Table 8-2.

IV. INSOMNIA

  A. Insomnia is difficulty **falling asleep or staying asleep** that occurs three times per week for at least 1 month and leads to sleepiness during the day or causes problems fulfilling social or occupational obligations.

  B. Insomnia is associated with **anxiety** and may be an early sign of the onset of a severe depressive or psychotic episode.

  C. Patients must be screened for use of (or withdrawal from) common substances (e.g., **caffeine, alcohol,** benzodiazepines).

  D. Some people who claim to have insomnia are sedative abusers seeking drugs.

Table 8-2.
Major Sleep Disorders

Disorder (Occurrence in the General Population)	Patient Snapshot	Etiology	Treatment
Insomnia (30%)	A 28-year-old man says that most nights during the last year he has lain awake in bed for more than 2 hours before he falls asleep. His sleep is often interrupted. The next day, he is tired and forgetful and often makes mistakes in his work.	Physiologic causes include medical conditions (e.g., pain, endocrine and metabolic diseases), substance use (especially caffeine) and withdrawal; the most common psychological etiologies are anxiety and depressive disorders	Avoidance of caffeine before bedtime; daily exercise (but not just before sleep); development of a series of behaviors associated with bedtime (i.e., "sleep ritual" or "sleep hygiene"); relaxation techniques; time-limited use of sleep agents establish an effective sleep pattern (e.g., zolpidem 10 mg at bedtime for 1–2 weeks); antidepressants or antipsychotics (if appropriate)
Narcolepsy (0.02%–0.16%)	A 22-year-old medical student who goes to sleep at 11 P.M. and wakes at 7 A.M., falls asleep in lab every day. She has had a few minor car accidents that occurred because she fell asleep while driving.	Usually starts in the late teens or early twenties; may have a genetic component	Stimulant drugs [e.g., methylphenidate (Ritalin), 10–60 mg daily for adults (if cataplexy is present, antidepressants may be added)]; modafinil (Provigil), 200 mg once daily; timed daytime naps may also be also useful
Breathing-related sleep disorder (obstructive sleep apnea) (1%–10%)	An overweight 55-year-old man reports that he is sleepy all day despite having 8 hours of sleep each night. His wife reports that his loud snoring keeps her awake.	Upper-airway obstruction (obstructive sleep apnea); may have a genetic component	Weight loss (first choice if appropriate); continuous positive airway pressure (CPAP); uvulopalatoplasty or tracheostomy (as a last resort)

V. NARCOLEPSY

    A. Patients with narcolepsy have **sleep attacks** (i.e., fall asleep suddenly during the day) despite having a normal amount of sleep at night.

B. Narcolepsy is also characterized by:

1. Hypnagogic or hypnopompic hallucinations, which occur just as the patient falls asleep or wakes up, respectively (20%–40% of patients)

2. Short REM latency

3. Cataplexy, or sudden physical collapse because of loss of all muscle tone after a strong emotional stimulus (70% of patients)

4. Sleep paralysis, in which the body is paralyzed for a few seconds after waking (30%–50% of patients)

C. Narcolepsy occurs most frequently in **adolescents and young adults.**

D. The **differential diagnosis** includes sleep deprivation, sleep apnea leading to daytime sleepiness, abuse of sedative drugs, and withdrawal from stimulant drugs.

VI. BREATHING-RELATED SLEEP DISORDER (SLEEP APNEA)

A. Patients with sleep apnea **stop breathing briefly.** Low oxygen or high carbon dioxide level in the blood awakens the patient repeatedly during the night, resulting in daytime sleepiness.

1. In patients with **central sleep apnea** (more common in the elderly), little or no respiratory effort occurs.

2. In patients with **obstructive sleep apnea,** which is more common in men (8:1, male to female ratio), in people 40–60 years old, and in the **obese,** respiratory effort occurs, but an airway obstruction prevents air from reaching the lungs. Patients often snore.

B. The **differential diagnosis** includes narcolepsy, depression-related hypersomnia, nocturnal panic attacks, use of sedative drugs, and withdrawal from stimulant drugs.

C. Sleep apnea is related to **depression, headaches,** and **pulmonary hypertension,** and also may result in **sudden death** during sleep in the elderly and in infants.

VII. OTHER SLEEP DISORDERS

A. Sleep terror disorder is the repetitive experience of fright in which a person (usually a child) screams in fear.

1. Sleep terrors **occur during delta (slow-wave) sleep.** The child's eyes may be open but he cannot be awakened and cannot remember the experience the next day.

2. Sleep terrors that begin in adolescence may indicate **temporal lobe epilepsy.**

B. Nightmare disorder is characterized by repetitive, frightening dreams that cause nighttime awakenings. It occurs during **REM sleep,** and the person usually can recall the nightmare.

C. Sleepwalking disorder begins in childhood (usually 4–8 years of age). The person walks around without being conscious and does not remember the episode. Sleepwalking is repetitive and occurs during delta (slow-wave) sleep.

D. Circadian rhythm sleep disorder causes a pattern of sleeping and waking at inappropriate times.

E. Nocturnal myoclonus and restless leg syndrome are repetitive muscular contractions in the legs and frequent motion of the legs, respectively. Both may cause nighttime awakening and are commonly treated with clonazepam (0.5–2 mg in divided doses).

F. **Kleine-Levin syndrome** is a rare condition that primarily affects adolescent boys. It causes recurrent periods of hypersomnia and hyperphagia (overeating), each lasting 1–3 weeks.

G. **Sleep drunkenness** is repetitive difficulty fully awakening after adequate sleep. It is associated with genetic factors.

H. **Menstrual-associated syndrome** is characterized by hypersomnia and hyperphagia occurring in the premenstrual period.

9
Cognitive Disorders

I. OVERVIEW

A. Characteristics

    1. The hallmarks of cognitive disorders (formerly called "organic mental syndromes") are **cognitive problems,** such as deficits in memory, orientation, judgment, or mental function.

    2. Mood changes, anxiety, irritability, paranoia, and psychosis, if present, occur as a result of the cognitive loss.

    3. The major cognitive disorders are:

        a. Delirium
        b. Dementia
        c. Amnestic disorder

B. Etiology

    1. Cognitive disorders are caused primarily by abnormalities in the **chemistry, structure, or physiology** of the brain.

    2. The underlying problem may originate in the brain, or the disorder may be secondary to systemic illness.

II. DELIRIUM

A. Characteristics

    1. Delirium is characterized by **clouding of consciousness, fluctuating course with lucid intervals,** and difficulty with orientation and attention due to **central nervous system dysfunction.**

    2. The patient first loses orientation to time, then to place, and, finally, to person.

    3. The patient appears hyperactive or hypoactive, **anxious, and confused.** Sleep disturbances, sleep reversals, and autonomic dysfunction are common.

B. Occurrence

    1. Delirium has many causes and is the **most common psychiatric syndrome** in hospitalized patients, particularly those in **surgical and coronary intensive care units.**

    2. Delirium is more common in **children, elderly people,** and patients with **preexisting brain damage.**

    3. Delirium usually occurs during an acute medical illness in a patient with no history of psychiatric illness.

C. Differential diagnosis and etiology

    1. Conditions that mimic delirium include dementia, psychosis, and depression.

    2. Delirium is one of the only psychiatric disorders in which the EEG is abnormal, showing fast wave activity or generalized slowing.

    3. The four **most common causes** of delirium are:

        a. Diseases of and injuries to the **central nervous system** (e.g., meningitis, head trauma)

        b. **Systemic illness** (e.g., liver, kidney, cardiovascular, or lung disease)

        c. **Drug abuse** (e.g., phencyclidine, sedatives, alcohol)

        d. **Drug withdrawal,** particularly from sedatives (e.g., alcohol, benzodiazepines, barbiturates)

    4. Other causes include fever, sensory deprivation, postoperative conditions, and medications, especially drug classes such as **anticholinergics.**

D. Prognosis

    1. The prognosis is good if the underlying medical cause can be treated effectively.

    2. Untreated delirium can progress to **dementia or death.**

III. DEMENTIA

A. Characteristics

    1. Cortical dementia is characterized by **gradual loss of memory and intellectual abilities** and has many causes. Symptoms that develop later in the illness include confusion and psychosis that progress to coma and death.

    2. **Subcortical dementia** [seen in Huntington disease, Parkinson disease, and human immunodeficiency virus (HIV) encephalopathy] is characterized by affective instability and movement disorders.

    3. Secondary emotional symptoms (e.g., anxiety, depression) are commonly seen in the early stages of dementia.

    4. The **distinction between delirium and dementia** is important (Table 9-1) because delirium often can be treated effectively.

B. Occurrence

    1. Dementia is **most commonly seen in the elderly.** At least 20% of people older than 80 years of age have significant dementia.

    2. In one-half to two-thirds of patients, the disorder is **dementia of the Alzheimer type.** Women are at slightly higher risk than men.

    3. The next most common type (15%–30%) is **vascular dementia** (formerly called "multi-infarct dementia").

C. Etiology

    1. The etiology of dementia of the Alzheimer type is unknown. However, gross and microscopic **neuroanatomic, neurophysiologic, genetic, and neurotransmitter** factors have been implicated (Table 9-2).

    2. In addition to vascular dementia, other causes of dementia are Lewy body disease, metastatic or primary tumor, Huntington disease, Parkinson disease, head trauma, multiple sclerosis, Creutzfeldt-Jakob disease, and Pick disease.

Table 9-1.
Comparison of Delirium and Dementia

Delirium Hallmark: impaired consciousness	Dementia Hallmark: loss of memory and intellectual abilities
(PATIENT SNAPSHOT) One week after an acute myocardial infarction, a 56-year-old man with no history of psychiatric illness becomes agitated and reports seeing strange animals in his room.	*(PATIENT SNAPSHOT)* A 72-year-old retired legal secretary is alert, but shows noticeable memory disturbance and does not know what day it is, nor can she precisely identify the woman next to her (her daughter).
Consciousness impaired or clouded	Consciousness not impaired
Develops quickly	Develops slowly
Fluctuations and lucid intervals	Steady course
Stupor or agitation	Normal level of arousal
Illusions or hallucinations, often visual	Illusions or hallucinations uncommon
Associated primarily with anxiety	Associated primarily with depression
Autonomic dysfunction	Little autonomic dysfunction
Diurnal variability, worse at night (i.e., "sundowning")	Little diurnal variability
EEG fast wave activity or generalized slowing	EEG usually normal
Frequently reversible if the underlying medical cause is removed	Reversible with treatment in a minority of cases, depending on the cause; pharmacotherapy is used for associated psychiatric symptoms

Table 9-2.
Pathophysiology of Dementia of the Alzheimer Type

Gross Neuroanatomy	Microscopic Neuroanatomy	Neurophysiology	Genetic Associations	Neurotransmitter Relations
• Enlarged brain ventricles • Diffuse atrophy • Flattened sulci	• Senile (amyloid) plaques and neurofibrillary tangles (seen also in Down syndrome and, to a lesser degree, in normal aging) • Loss of cholinergic neurons in the basal forebrain • Neuronal loss and degeneration in the hippocampus and cortex	• Reduction in brain levels of choline acetyltransferase (needed to synthesize acetylcholine) • Abnormal processing of amyloid precursor protein. • Decreased membrane fluidity because of abnormal regulation of membrane phospholipid metabolism	• Abnormalities of chromosomes 1, 14, and 21 (as in Down syndrome) • Possession of at least one copy of the apo E_4 gene on chromosome 19 • Having a close relative with dementia of the Alzheimer type	• Decreased activity of acetylcholine and norepinephrine. • Abnormal activity of somatostatin, vasoactive intestinal peptide, and corticotropin

3. **HIV infection** often leads to dementia.

    a. HIV can infect the brain directly, causing atrophy, inflammation, and demyelination. Dementia can also result from cerebral lymphoma or opportunistic brain infection in HIV-infected patients.

    b. Death occurs within 6 months in most patients with HIV dementia.

D. **Dementia of the Alzheimer type**

    1. Characteristics and occurrence

        a. Normal consciousness despite severe **memory loss and language difficulties** (see patient snapshot under "Dementia" in Table 9-1)

        b. **Changes in personality** (e.g., anger, paranoia) and mood (e.g., depression)

        c. **Slow onset and progressive deterioration** in cognitive function

    2. Differential diagnosis

        a. Normal aging is associated with reduction in the ability to learn new things quickly and a general slowing of mental processes. In contrast to dementia of the Alzheimer type, **changes associated with normal aging** do not interfere with normal functioning.

        b. Dementia of the Alzheimer type is **commonly confused with depression** ("pseudodementia"), which can mimic cognitive impairment, but which responds to treatment with antidepressant agents (see Chapter 13).

    3. Treatment

        a. **Psychosocial** treatment includes providing a **structured environment,** a nutritious diet, exercise, and recreational therapy for the patient as well as supportive psychotherapy and support groups for family caregivers.

        b. **Pharmacologic** treatment includes antianxiety, antidepressant, and antipsychotic agents to relieve associated symptoms.

        c. **Tacrine** (Cognex), a cholinesterase inhibitor, improves cognitive function transiently but may cause adverse effects, including elevated liver enzyme levels and gastrointestinal disturbances. Newer cholinesterase inhibitors **donepezil** (Aricept), **rivastigmine** (Exelor), and **galantamine** (Reminyl) may be more effective and have fewer side effects.

    4. Prognosis

        a. **Memory** is affected first (recent memory before remote memory), followed by language (e.g., difficulty finding the right word), then spatial ability (e.g., difficulty copying a simple drawing).

        b. **Life expectancy** is approximately **8 years after diagnosis.**

E. Vascular dementias

    1. Characteristics

        a. A 75-year-old man with no history of psychiatric disorder suddenly cannot remember what to do when the telephone rings or how to turn on the microwave oven.

        b. Men are at higher risk than women.

        c. In contrast to dementia of the Alzheimer type, vascular dementias are associated with:

            (1) **Sudden,** rather than gradual, onset of cognitive dysfunction

            (2) **Stepwise,** rather than steady, deterioration of function

            (3) Less deterioration of the patient's personality characteristics

(4) Focal neurologic symptoms

2. Etiology

   a. Multiple small cerebral infarctions occur as a result of atherosclerosis, hypertension, valvular heart disease, or arrhythmias.

   b. Each infarct causes an abrupt loss of function.

3. Treatment to decrease the likelihood of repeated infarcts includes reducing the risk factors associated with cardiovascular disease (i.e., hypertension, excessive body weight, smoking, alcohol abuse, arrhythmias).

F. **Amnestic disorder**

   1. Characteristics

   a. An alert 56-year-old man with a superficially jovial affect has a 30-year history of alcoholism. He claims that he was drafted into the army in 1999.

   b. **Memory loss** occurs, with little other cognitive impairment and a normal level of consciousness.

   c. Both retrograde amnesia (i.e., memory for past events, particularly the recent past) and anterograde amnesia (i.e., inability to put down new memories) occur; the patient may fabricate forgotten information to cover memory loss **(confabulation).**

   2. The **differential diagnosis** includes dementia, delirium, normal aging, dissociative disorders, and factitious disorder (see Chapter 15).

   3. Etiology, treatment, and prognosis

   a. The primary cause of amnestic disorder is **thiamine deficiency** as a result of **long-term alcohol abuse (Korsakoff syndrome).** Korsakoff syndrome often follows an episode of **Wernicke's encephalopathy,** an acute condition with multiple neurological signs. The thiamine deficiency contributes to **destruction of mediotemporal lobe structures** (e.g., mammillary bodies, hippocampus, fornix).

   b. Other causes of amnestic disorder include head injury, cerebrovascular disease or infection involving the temporal lobes (e.g., herpes simplex encephalitis), and exposure to neurotoxins.

   c. Treatment and prognosis depend on the underlying cause.

10
Substance-Related Disorders

I. SUBSTANCE ABUSE, TOLERANCE, AND DEPENDENCE

A. Definitions

    1. **Substance abuse** is a pattern of abnormal drug use that leads to **impairment** of social, physical, or occupational functioning.

    2. **Substance dependence** is substance abuse plus **tolerance, withdrawal,** or a pattern of **compulsive use.**

        a. **Tolerance** is the need for **increased amounts** of the substance to achieve the same positive effects.

        b. **Cross-tolerance** is the development of tolerance to one substance as the result of using another substance.

        c. **Withdrawal** is the development of psychological or physical symptoms after the reduction or cessation of intake of a substance.

B. Common psychiatric syndromes associated with substance abuse include mood disorders, anxiety disorders, borderline and antisocial personality disorders, schizophrenia, and conduct disorder in adolescents.

II. CLASSES OF ABUSED SUBSTANCES

A. **Stimulants** are central nervous system activators that include caffeine, nicotine, cocaine, and amphetamines.

    1. Amphetamines are used clinically to treat attention-deficit/hyperactivity disorder (ADHD), narcolepsy, and refractory depression.

    2. The most commonly used amphetamines are dextroamphetamine (Dexedrine), methamphetamine (Desoxyn), and a related compound, methylphenidate (Ritalin).

    3. "Speed," "ice" (methamphetamine), and "ecstasy" (MDMA or methylene dioxymethamphetamine) are street names for amphetamine compounds.

    4. "Crack" and "freebase" are smokable forms of cocaine.

B. **Sedatives are central nervous system depressants** that include alcohol, barbiturates, and benzodiazepines.

C. **Narcotics** are drugs in the **opioid** class, which includes pharmaceuticals (e.g., morphine, codeine) and drugs of abuse (e.g., heroin).

D. **Hallucinogens** include lysergic acid diethylamide (LSD), cannabis (tetrahydrocannabinol, marijuana, hashish), psilocybin (from mushrooms), and mescaline (from

Table 10-1.
Epidemiology of Commonly Used Substances

Substance	Used Drug in Last Year/ Used Drug in Lifetime*	Comments
Caffeine	75%/80%	Most commonly used psychoactive drug; found in coffee (125 mg/cup), tea (65 mg/cup), cola (40 mg/cup), nonprescription stimulants, and diet agents
Alcohol	50%/85%	10%–13% lifetime prevalence of abuse or dependence; male:female ratio of at least 2:1; more serious health effects in women; increased use in Native Americans and Eskimos, in the 21- to 34-year-old age-group, correlated with childhood attention-deficit/ hyperactivity disorder and conduct disorder
Nicotine	30%/55%	Increased use in women, adolescents, and African-American adults, but decreased use in African-American adolescents; female smokers outnumber male smokers and experience more serious health effects; smoking decreases life expectancy more than the use of any other substance
Marijuana	10%/33%	Use is higher in the 18- to 25-year-old age group; most commonly used illegal psychoactive drug; use is increasing among adolescents; at least two states permit limited medical use to treat glaucoma and cancer-related nausea and vomiting
Cocaine	3%/12%	Primarily used by people in lower social economic groups in its inexpensive crack form (smoked); also used by people in higher socioeconomic groups in its expensive, pure form (snorted into the nose); use is declining
Amphetamines	1.3%/7%	High-risk groups include professionals, people who work late at night (e.g., musicians, students), and 18- to 25-year-olds
Heroin	0.2%/1.3%	Male:female ratio of 3:1

*These numbers are conservative estimates.

cactus). Phencyclidine (PCP, "angel dust") has effects similar to LSD but is pharmacologically in a different category.

III. **EPIDEMIOLOGY AND DEMOGRAPHICS.** Caffeine, nicotine, alcohol, and marijuana and, to a lesser extent, cocaine, amphetamines and heroin, are the **most commonly abused substances** in the United States (Table 10-1).

IV. **CLINICAL FEATURES**

A. Substances produce **physical and psychological signs and symptoms** that indicate use. They also cause characteristic **withdrawal symptoms** (Table 10-2).

B. **Laboratory findings** can usually confirm substance use (Table 10-3).

C. Certain **neurotransmitter systems** are associated with the use of specific substances.

1. **Increased** availability of **dopamine** (DA) is associated with the effects of **stimulants** and **opiates.**

a. Amphetamine use causes the release of DA. Cocaine blocks the reuptake of DA.

Table 10-2.

Signs, Symptoms and Complications of Drug Abuse

Type	Substance	Effects of Use	Withdrawal Symptoms
Stimulants	Amphetamines Cocaine	Euphoria, loss of appetite, fever, tachycardia, psychotic symptoms, including tactile hallucinations (with cocaine), dilated pupils. Amphetamines are medically indicated for attention deficit hyperactivity disorder in children, narcolepsy, refractory depression, and short-term treatment of obesity (usually of an amphetamine-like drug, such as phentermine) if state laws permit	Post-use "crash," including depression, malaise, fatigue, hunger, psychological craving for the drug, and constricted pupils
	Caffeine Nicotine	Agitation, insomnia, increased peristalsis, vasoconstriction of peripheral blood vessels, cardiac arrhythmias	Headache, slight weight gain, lethargy, depression
Sedatives	Alcohol	Elevated mood followed by depression, liver dysfunction (e.g., cirrhosis), gastrointestinal symptoms (e.g., ulcers), thiamine deficiency (resulting in Wernicke and Korsakoff syndromes), fetal alcohol syndrome, reduced life expectancy; associated with disinhibition, traffic fatalities, suicide, rape, assault, and homicide	Anxiety; tremor; delirium tremens, including tactile hallucinations (e.g., formication or sensation of ants crawling on the skin); seizures; withdrawal may be life-threatening; hospitalization is usually required
	Barbiturates Benzodiazepines	Respiratory depression; high suicide potential; high addiction potential Respiratory depression when combined with alcohol; moderately high addiction potential	Anxiety, tremor, seizures, withdrawal may be life-threatening; hospitalization is usually required
Narcotics	Opiates	Euphoria, respiratory depression, hypothermia, hypotension, constricted pupils (miosis)	Anxiety, sweating, fever, runny nose (rhinorrhea), goose bumps (piloerection), tearing (lacrimation), nausea, stomach cramps, dilated pupils (mydriasis), yawning; uncomfortable, but rarely life-threatening

(*continued*)

Table 10-2.—*Continued*

Signs, Symptoms and Complications of Drug Abuse

Type	Substance	Effects of Use	Withdrawal Symptoms
Hallucinogens and related agents	Lysergic acid diethylamide (LSD)	Effects last 8–12 hours and include profuse perspiration, blurred vision, dilated pupils, tachycardia, tremor, palpitations, and altered perception and emotions; long-term cognitive impairment; "bad trips" (i.e., panic reactions that may include psychotic symptoms); "flashbacks" (i.e., a reexperience of the associated sensations in the absence of the drug)	No significant withdrawal symptoms
	Phencyclidine "angel dust" (PCP)	Hypertension, hyperthermia, horizontal and vertical nystagmus (abnormal eye movements); fantasies, euphoria, amnesia, episodes of extremely violent behavior; auditory and visual hallucinations; distortions of body image, time, and space; aggressiveness; consumption greater than 20 mg may cause convulsions, coma, and death; long-term effects include memory loss, lethargy and reduced attention span	No significant withdrawal symptoms
	Marijuana	Low dose impairs memory and complex motor activity, alters sensory and time perception, causes conjunctival reddening, and may increase appetite and sexual desire; at high doses, causes psychotic symptoms and paranoia; chronic use causes decreased sexual functioning, lung problems associated with smoking, decreased motivation (i.e., the "amotivational" syndrome)	No significant withdrawal symptoms

   b. Both the release of DA and the blockade of DA reuptake result in increased availability of the neurotransmitter in the synapse.

   c. Increased availability of DA in the synapse is apparently involved in the "reward" system of the brain and the euphoric effects of stimulants and opiates.

2. **Increased** activity of the inhibitory neurotransmitter γ-aminobutyric acid **(GABA)** is associated with the effects of **sedative** agents.

3. **Increased** availability of **serotonin** is associated with the effects of some **hallucinogens.**

Table 10-3.
Laboratory Findings with Drugs of Abuse

Substance	Laboratory Findings
Alcohol	Elevated blood alcohol level (intoxication defined as blood alcohol level $> 0.08\%-0.15\%$, depending on state law); tolerance is likely if symptoms of intoxication are absent despite blood alcohol level of $> 0.10\%$; elevated (> 30 units) gamma-glutamyltransferase (GGT) level
Barbiturates Benzodiazepines	Specific sedatives or their metabolites can be identified in blood; urine test results are positive for as long as 1 week
Opiates	Most opiates are present in urine and blood for 12–36 hours after use; methadone can be detected for 2–3 days after use; fentanyl is not identified by common tests for opiates
Amphetamines	Present in urine for 1–2 days
Cocalne	Increased level of benzoylecgonine (metabolite) for 1–3 days in occasional users, 7–12 days in heavy users
Nicotine	Increased level of cotinine (metabolite) in urine, blood, and saliva
Lysergic acid diethylamide (LSD)	Urine toxicology results are positive for LSD
Phencyclidine, "angel dust" (PCP)	Present in urine for > 1 week; elevated serum glutamic-oxaloacetic transaminase (SGOT) level; elevated creatinine phosphokinase (CPK) level
Marijuana	Cannabinoid metabolites are present in urine for 7–10 days (as long as 28 days in heavy users)

V. TREATMENT

    A. Treatment of substance abuse ranges from abstinence and peer support groups to drugs that block withdrawal symptoms (Table 10-4).

    B. Dual diagnosis or **MICA (mentally ill–chemically addicted)** patients require treatment for both substance abuse and the co-morbid psychiatric illness (e.g. major depression), often on a special unit in the hospital.

Table 10-4.

Treatment of Abuse of Commonly Used Substances

Substance	Immediate Treatment	Long-term Treatment
Caffeine	Eliminate or taper from the diet (substitute decaffeinated beverage)	Analgesics to control headache caused by withdrawal
Nicotine	Nicotine-containing gum, patch, or nasal spray; support from a spouse, child, or nonsmoking physician	Peer support groups; most of those who quit on their own experience relapse within 2 years; the relapse rate among members of peer support groups is better; the antidepressant bupropion (Zyban) may help maintain abstinence
Alcohol	Thiamine 100 mg IM initially and 200 mg/day for 4 days; restore nutritional state Benzodiazepines are useful for withdrawal symptoms; for anxiety, chlordiazepoxide (25–100 mg) or diazepam (10–20 mg) every 4 hours; for delirium, dose every hour; for seizures, 100–150 mg phenobarbital IM or 5–10 mg diazepam IV	Alcoholics Anonymous (AA) or other peer support groups (12-step programs) are the most effective treatment; disulfiram [Antabuse] 125–500 mg/day, which causes an accumulation of acetaldehyde in the blood, resulting in a toxic reaction including intense nausea, headache, and flushing when the patient subsequently drinks alcohol, is effective for motivated patients; individual or group psychotherapy and family therapy may be useful, particularly if the spouse participates
Marijuana	Calm the patient by "talking him down," benzodiazepines (e.g., diazepam 10–15 mg)	Abstinence and education
Barbiturates and benzodiazepines	Hospitalization, prevent seizures by gradually reducing dosage and substituting long-acting barbiturates (e.g., phenobarbital) or benzodiazepines (e.g., diazepam) for the more commonly abused short-acting types; flumazenil (Romazicon 0.2 mg–3.0 mg) titrated intravenously as antidote for overdose	Psychological support, behavior therapy
Hallucinogens	Calm the patient by "talking her down," hospitalization and medical maintenance, benzodiazepines (e.g., diazepam, 10–20 mg orally) to decrease agitation, antipsychotics (e.g., haloperidol 5–10 mg IM or 10 mg orally) to treat psychotic symptoms	Education for initiation and maintenance of abstinence
Cocaine	Medical support to prevent or treat cardiac symptoms and seizures, benzodiazepines to treat agitation, antipsychotics to treat psychotic symptoms	Treatment of psychological withdrawal symptoms with desipramine (Norpramin 200–250 mg/day)

(continued)

Table 10-4.—*Continued*
Treatment of Abuse of Commonly Used Substances

Substance	Immediate Treatment	Long-term Treatment
Amphetamines	Benzodiazepines to treat agitation, antipsychotics to treat psychotic symptoms, medical and psychological support	No specific treatment has proven effective in the initiation and maintenance of abstinence
Heroin	For overdose, short-acting opioid antagonists; naloxone (Narcan) 0.4 mg IV, five doses at 3-minute intervals, more if needed Methadone detoxification (10 mg orally four times daily for 7 days) Clonidine (0.15 mg twice daily) helps in withdrawal by suppressing autonomic symptoms	Methadone maintenance: reduce to 10%–20% of detoxification dose when patient is stable; methadone is taken orally rather than injected, is less sedating, and has less euphoric action than heroin; it causes physical dependence and tolerance, but suppresses withdrawal symptoms, allowing the person to have a relatively normal life; L-methadyl acetate hydrochloride (LAAM) is a synthetic opioid agonist with a longer duration of action than methadone Naltrexone (Revia) can be used to maintain abstinence by blocking opiate receptors; voluntary peer support 12-step programs, such as Narcotics Anonymous, may be helpful

11

Schizophrenia

I. CHARACTERISTICS

A. A 28-year-old man who lives in a group home says that his roommates are spying on him by listening to him through the television set. For this reason, he has changed roommates a number of times over the last 5 years. He dresses strangely, is unkempt and dirty, and seems preoccupied by "people giving him instructions in his head."

B. Specific characteristics

    1. Schizophrenia is a **chronic, debilitating mental disorder** that is characterized by disturbed thought, behavior, and speech.

    2. The patient often has a strange appearance, shows poor grooming, and is socially withdrawn.

    3. In the psychotic phase, the patient shows a loss of touch with reality. In the prodromal and residual phases, despite many other symptoms, the patient is generally in touch with reality.

    4. The patient has an abnormal affect (i.e., inappropriate, flat, or blunted).

    5. The patient shows intact memory capacity and is oriented to person, place, and time.

C. DSM-IV-TR criteria

    1. Symptoms (prodromal, acute psychotic, and residual) that last for 6 months

    2. At least one period of actual psychosis within the 6-month period

    3. Impairment of occupational or social functioning during the 6-month period

D. Prodromal signs and symptoms

    1. Before the first psychotic episode, the patient often avoids social activities and makes few friends. He is usually quiet, passive, or irritable.

    2. The patient may also have physical complaints and show new interest in religion, the occult, or philosophy.

E. Psychotic signs and symptoms. Thought disorders and other characteristic clinical signs occur during an acute psychotic episode. Specific descriptions and examples are shown in Table 11-1. They include disorders of:

    1. Perception (e.g., hallucinations)

    2. Thought content (e.g., delusions, ideas of reference, loss of ego boundaries)

Table 11-1.
Signs and Symptoms of Psychosis

Sign or Symptom	Definition	Example
Hallucinations	False sensory perceptions; auditory hallucinations are most common; visual, tactile, gustatory, olfactory, and cenesthetic (visceral) hallucinations also occur	The patient hears two different voices holding a conversation about her when she is alone in a room. Sometimes she smells nonexistent odors.
Delusions	False beliefs that are not correctable by logic or reason, are not based on simple ignorance, and are not shared by a culture or subculture; delusions of persecution are most common	The patient believes that she is being followed by government agents who want to steal her secrets.
Ideas of reference	False belief that one is the subject of attention by other people or the media	The patient believes that she is being discussed on a national television program.
Loss of ego boundaries	Not knowing where one's mind and body end and those of others begin	The patient feels that she is "merged" into others.
Thought blocking	Abrupt halt in the train of thinking, often because of hallucinations	The patient suddenly stops talking, even though her lips are moving, and she seems to be concentrating on an inner stimulus.
Impaired abstraction ability	Difficulty in discerning the essential qualities of objects or relations despite normal intelligence	When asked what brought him to the hospital, the patient says "a car."
Neologisms	Inventing new words (without a conscious attempt at humor)	The patient refers to the psychiatrist as a "medicinal shrinkomat."
Word salad	Uttering unrelated combinations of words or phrases	The patient says, "I'm not so utterly pure that I'm going away anyway to break it."
Loose associations	Ideas shift from one subject to another in an unrelated or partially related fashion	The patient begins to answer a question about her job, then launches into a diatribe about capitalism.
Echolalia	Parroting words just spoken by another person	Doctor asks "Are you feeling sad?" Patient responds "Are you feeling sad?"
Tangentiality	Beginning a response in a logical fashion, but then getting further and further from the point	The patient says "I'll tell you about my headache, but let me tell you about other things in my head, like thoughts about God."
Perseveration	Repeating a thought over and over	The patient says, "I'm sane . . . I'm sane . . . I'm sane . . . that I'm sane."

3. Thought processes (e.g., thought blocking, impaired abstraction ability, neologisms)

4. Form of thought (e.g., word salad, loose associations, echolalia, tangentiality, perseveration)

F. Residual signs and symptoms. In schizophrenia, signs and symptoms that occur between episodes of acute psychosis are called "residual." They include:

    1. Flat or inappropriate affect (e.g., bland reaction to disturbing news)

    2. Peculiar thinking and eccentric behavior (e.g., reading personal meaning into natural phenomena)

    3. Social withdrawal (e.g., choosing to work the night shift in order to be alone)

G. Positive and negative symptoms. Symptoms of schizophrenia can also be classified as positive or negative. These classifications can be useful in predicting the effects of antipsychotic medication.

    1. Positive (productive) symptoms are characterized by "excessive" function.

        a. Positive symptoms include delusions, hallucinations, agitation, strange behavior, and talkativeness.

        b. These symptoms respond well to most traditional antipsychotic agents.

    2. Negative (deficit) symptoms are characterized by decreased function.

        a. Negative symptoms include flattened affect, thought blocking, cognitive disturbances, poor grooming, lack of motivation, social withdrawal, and impoverished speech content.

        b. Negative symptoms respond better to atypical agents, such as clozapine (Clozaril), risperidone (Risperdal), olanzapine (Zyprexa), quetiapine (Seroquel), and ziprasidone (Geodon) than to traditional antipsychotics.

II. SUBTYPES. DSM-IV-TR lists five subtypes of schizophrenia (Table 11-2).

III. DIFFERENTIAL DIAGNOSIS

    A. Medical illnesses that may mimic schizophrenia include neurologic disease or head trauma, temporal lobe epilepsy, early dementia, delirium, poisoning, and endocrine disorders (psychotic disorder caused by a general medical condition).

    B. Psychiatric illnesses that mimic schizophrenia include brief psychotic disorder, schizophreniform disorder, schizoaffective disorder, delusional disorder, the manic phase of bipolar disorder, severe personality disorders (e.g., schizoid, schizotypal, borderline), and substance-induced psychotic disorder (Table 11-3).

Table 11-2.
DSM-IV-TR Subtypes of Schizophrenia

Subtype (Most Common to Least Common)	Characteristics
Undifferentiated	Characteristics of more than one subtype
Paranoid	Delusions of persecution; older age of onset and better functioning than other subtypes
Residual	One previous schizophrenic episode; subsequently shows residual symptoms, but no psychotic symptoms
Disorganized (hebephrenic)	Disinhibition; poor organization, personal appearance, and grooming; inappropriate emotional responses; age of onset before 25 years
Catatonic	Bizarre posturing (waxy flexibility), muteness, stupor or extreme excitability; rare since the introduction of antipsychotic agents

Table 11-3.
Differential Diagnoses of Schizophrenia

Disorder	Distinguishing Characteristics
Psychotic disorder due to a general medical condition	Clouding of consciousness; hallucinations are visual condition and changeable rather than auditory and recurrent; occurs in the context of an acute medical illness
Brief psychotic disorder	Psychotic and residual symptoms lasting > 1 day but < 1 month; often obvious precipitating psychosocial factors
Schizophreniform disorder	Psychotic and residual symptoms lasting 1–6 months (for schizophrenia, symptoms last > 6 months)
Schizoaffective disorder	Symptoms of a major mood disorder as well as of schizophrenia; chronic social and occupational impairment
Manic episode in bipolar disorder	Psychotic symptoms, elated mood, hyperactivity, rapid speech, sociability; rapid onset; little or no impairment in social or occupational functioning between episodes
Delusional disorder	Fixed, long-lasting nonbizarre delusional system; few, if any, other thought disorders; relatively normal social and occupational functioning
Schizoid personality disorder	Social withdrawal without psychosis
Schizotypal personality disorder	Peculiar behavior and odd thought patterns, such as magical thinking (e.g., the idea that wishing can make something happen), without psychosis
Borderline personality disorder	Extreme mood swings, with uncontrollable anger, dissociation, and episodic suicidal thoughts; minipsychotic episodes (lasting only minutes)
Substance-induced psychotic disorder	Prominent hallucinations (often visual or tactile) or delusions directly related to the use or withdrawal of a specific drug (especially amphetamines, hallucinogens, and alcohol); (see Chapter 10)

IV. OCCURRENCE

    A. Risk of schizophrenia

        1. 50% for monozygotic twins of patients with schizophrenia

        2. 40% for people with two parents with schizophrenia

        3. 12% for first-degree relatives (i.e., child, sibling) of people with schizophrenia

        4. 1% for the general population

    B. Age of onset, sex, and race

        1. Peak age of onset of schizophrenia is 15–25 years of age for men and 25–35 years of age for women. In 90% of patients, first onset occurs at 15–45 years of age. Schizophrenia is rarely diagnosed if the initial episode occurs after 45 years of age.

        2. Schizophrenia occurs **equally in men and women** and in all cultures and ethnic groups studied.

C. Seasonal factors. More people with schizophrenia are **born during cold weather months** (i.e., January through April in the northern hemisphere and July through September in the southern hemisphere). One possible explanation for this finding is viral infection of the mother during the second trimester of pregnancy, since infections occur seasonally.

V. ETIOLOGY

A. Neural pathology

1. Abnormalities of the frontal lobes, as evidenced by decreased use of glucose in the frontal lobes on positron emission tomography (PET) scans

2. Lateral and third ventricle enlargement, abnormal cerebral symmetry, and changes in brain density

3. Decreased size of the hippocampus, amygdala, and parahippocampal gyrus

4. Possible involvement of the basal ganglia (because movement problems occur in some patients)

B. Neurotransmitter abnormalities

1. The dopamine hypothesis of schizophrenia states that schizophrenia results from **excessive dopaminergic activity** (e.g., excessive number of dopamine receptors, excessive concentration of dopamine, hypersensitivity of receptors to dopamine). Laboratory tests may show **elevated levels of homovanillic acid,** a metabolite of dopamine, in body fluids.

2. Serotonin hyperactivity is implicated in schizophrenia because hallucinogens that increase serotonin levels cause psychotic symptoms and because most effective atypical antipsychotics have anti-serotonergic-2 (5-HT_2) activity.

3. Norepinephrine hyperactivity is implicated, particularly in paranoid schizophrenia.

4. γ-Aminobutyric acid (GABA) is implicated because patients with schizophrenia show loss of **GABA-ergic neurons** in the hippocampus.

C. Abnormal clinical findings

1. Electroencephalogram (EEG) findings show decreased alpha waves, increased theta and delta waves, and epileptiform activity.

2. Eye movements (e.g., poor smooth visual pursuit) are abnormal in 50%–80% of schizophrenic patients as well as in unaffected relatives.

3. Neuroendocrine abnormalities, such as decreased levels of luteinizing hormone and follicle-stimulating hormone and abnormal regulation of cortisol, as demonstrated by positive dexamethasone suppression tests (see Chapter 3), are seen in some patients.

D. Social and environmental etiology

1. No social or environmental factor causes schizophrenia. However, because patients with schizophrenia tend to drift down the socioeconomic scale as a result of their social deficits (the **"downward drift"** hypothesis), they are often found in lower socioeconomic groups (e.g., homeless people).

2. Internal or external stress may shorten the time to onset or increase the severity of symptoms (the "stress diathesis" model) in schizophrenia.

VI. TREATMENT

A. Pharmacologic and psychological treatment

1. Pharmacologic treatments for schizophrenia include traditional antipsychotics [**dopamine-2 (D$_2$)-receptor antagonists**] and atypical antipsychotic agents (see Chapter 25). Atypicals have recently become first-line agents.

2. Psychological treatments, including individual, family, and group psychotherapy, are useful to provide long-term support and maintain compliance with the drug regimen.

B. Traditional antipsychotic agents

1. Traditional antipsychotic agents such as chlorpromazine (Thorazine) and haloperidol (Haldol) work primarily by blocking central D$_2$ receptors.

2. Significant improvement is seen in 70% of patients who take traditional antipsychotic agents (25% of these improvements occur as a result of the placebo effect). These agents are particularly effective against positive symptoms.

C. Atypical antipsychotic agents

3. Clozapine, an atypical antipsychotic, is a **D$_4$-receptor antagonist** that also acts on the serotonergic system.

    a. Clozapine is less likely to cause extrapyramidal symptoms (pseudo-parkinsonism, dystonias, akathisia), tardive dyskinesia, and neuroleptic malignant syndrome than traditional agents.

    b. Clozapine is **more likely to cause agranulocytosis, seizures, and anticholinergic side effects** than are traditional agents.

2. Other atypical antipsychotics, such as risperidone, olanzapine, quetiapine, and ziprasidone, have **anti-5-HT$_2$** as well as antidopaminergic receptor activity and cause fewer neurologic and hematologic side effects than clozapine.

D. Side effects of antipsychotic agents (Table 11-4)

1. **High-potency** antipsychotics such as haloperidol have primarily **neurologic side effects,** such as extrapyramidal symptoms, tardive dyskinesia, and neuroleptic malignant syndrome.

2. **Low-potency** antipsychotic agents such as chlorpromazine have primarily **anticholinergic and antihistaminic side effects.**

3. Other side effects of antipsychotics

    a. Cardiovascular problems, including electrocardiogram abnormalities and orthostatic hypotension

    b. **Weight gain and sedation,** especially with clozapine and olanzapine

    c. Hepatic effects, including jaundice and elevated liver enzyme levels

    d. Endocrine problems, primarily because of **increased levels of prolactin** that lead to gynecomastia, galactorrhea, impotence, amenorrhea, and decreased libido

    e. Hematologic dysfunction, including **leukopenia, agranulocytosis** (deficiency in some white blood cells, particularly polymorphonuclear leukocytes), especially with clozapine

    f. Dermatologic effects, including photosensitivity, skin eruptions, and blue-gray skin discoloration with chlorpromazine

    g. Ophthalmologic effects, including **irreversible retinal pigmentation caused**

Table 11-4.
Side Effects of Antipsychotic Medications and Their Treatment

Side Effect	Examples	Treatment
Extrapyramidal symptoms: Pseudoparkinsonism	Resting ("pill rolling") tremor, akinesia (slowed movements), and rigidity	Reduce dose of antipsychotic agent; give anticholinergic agents, e.g., amantadine (Symmetrel 100–200 mg/day), benztropine (Cogentin 1–4 mg/day), trihexyphenidyl (Artane 2–5 mg/day), or diphenhydramine (Benadryl 25–50 mg/day)
Acute dystonia	Slow, prolonged muscular spasms (most common in men younger than 40 years of age)	
Akathisia	Subjective feeling of motor restlessness	
Anticholinergic effects: Peripheral	Dry mouth, blurred vision, constipation, urinary retention	Salivary stimulants, physostigmine eye drops, stool softeners, and hydration, respectively
Central	Severe agitation and confusion	Physostigmine (Antilirium 1–2 mg IM or IV) repeated in 30 minutes
Tardive dyskinesia	Writhing, choreothetoid movements of the tongue, head, face, and mouth; more common in older women; usually occurs after 6 months of antipsychotic treatment; spontaneously remits in 50% of cases, but may be permanent	Symptoms often remit after discontinuation of traditional antipsychotics and substitution of an atypical agent; treatments that have been used with modest success include benzodiazepines, propranolol, and cholinomimetics (e.g., choline chloride)
Neuroleptic malignant syndrome	High fever, sweating, confusion, increased blood pressure and pulse, muscular rigidity, high creatine phosphokinase concentration, renal failure; more common in men and early in the treatment program; 20% mortality rate; medical emergency	Immediately discontinue antipsychotic agents; supportive medical treatment includes cooling the patient and hydration, dantrolene sodium (Dantrium up to 10 mg/kg/day IV); bromocriptine (Parlodel), and amantadine (Symmetrel) are also useful

by thioridazine (Mellaril) and deposits in the lens and cornea caused by chlorpromazine

4. Treatment of noncompliant patients includes long-acting injectable depot forms, such as fluphenazine (Prolixin) decanoate and haloperidol decanoate, which are administered intramuscularly every 4 weeks.

VII. COURSE AND PROGNOSIS

A. Course

1. Increasing agitation, depression, and insomnia indicate that a patient will have a psychotic episode.

2. Schizophrenia often involves repeated psychotic episodes and a chronic, downhill course. The illness often stabilizes in midlife.

3. During an acute psychotic episode, suicide may result from "command" hallucinations (i.e., a voice telling the patient to kill himself).

4. After the acute psychotic episode ends, post-psychotic depression occurs in 50% of patients. The patient may attempt **suicide.**

B. Prognosis

1. **Impairment is commonly lifelong.**

2. The prognosis is better if the patient is older at onset, is married or has social relationships, has mood symptoms, is female, has a good employment history, has positive symptoms, and has few relapses.

12

Other Psychotic Disorders

I. OVERVIEW

A. **Psychotic disorders** are all characterized at some point during their course by a gross impairment in reality testing. Schizophrenia (Chapter 11) is the most comprehensive model for a psychotic disorder. The following other psychotic disorders do not include all of the criteria required for the diagnosis of schizophrenia (Table 12-1).

   1. Brief psychotic disorder

   2. Schizophreniform disorder

   3. Schizoaffective disorder

   4. Delusional disorder

   5. Shared psychotic disorder (folie à deux)

B. **Differential diagnosis.** The differential diagnosis of schizophrenia also includes:

   1. The manic phase of bipolar disorder (see Chapter 13)

   2. Schizotypal, schizoid, paranoid, and borderline personality disorders (see Chapter 21)

C. Some mental disorders characterized by psychotic symptoms have an obvious **medical cause.** These disorders (formerly called "organic mental syndromes") include:

   1. Delirium, dementia, and amnestic and other cognitive disorders (see Chapter 9).

   2. Psychotic disorder due to a general medical condition (see Chapters 22 and 23).

   3. Substance-induced psychotic disorder (see Chapter 10).

II. TREATMENT AND PROGNOSIS. The treatment and prognosis of the other psychotic disorders are shown in Table 12-2.

Table 12-1.
Other Psychotic Disorders

Disorder	Patient Snapshot	Characteristics	Differences from Schizophrenia
Brief psychotic disorder	A 22-year-old man whose sister recently died of cancer is brought to the emergency room by his girlfriend. She reports that during the last 2 weeks, he has begun to show bizarre behavior and claims that he hears his sister talking to him.	Psychotic and residual symptoms lasting > 1 day but < 1 month; often precipitated by psychosocial factors; more common in patients with concomitant borderline and histrionic personality disorders	Much shorter duration of symptoms; relatively normal premorbid functioning, sudden onset and termination of symptoms; no family history of schizophrenia
Schizophreniform disorder	A 28-year-old woman with no history of psychiatric illness is brought to the emergency room by her husband. He says that approximately 2 months ago, she suddenly began to behave strangely and frequently seems preoccupied (as though she is listening to something).	Two or more psychotic symptoms as well as residual symptoms lasting at least 1 month but < 6 months	Shorter duration of symptoms; impairment of social or occupational functioning are not necessary for the diagnosis
Schizoaffective disorder	A 45-year-old man with a history of severe depression and psychotic symptoms has held different jobs, none of them for longer than 6 months. He is successfully treated for his severe depressive symptoms, but he remains psychotic and withdrawn.	Fits the criteria for both major mood disorder (mania or depression) and schizophrenia	Prominent affective (mood) symptoms

(continued)

Table 12-1.—*Continued*
Other Psychotic Disorders

Disorder	Patient Snapshot	Characteristics	Differences from Schizophrenia
Delusional disorder	A 68-year-old patient says that her neighbor has been trying to get her evicted from her apartment for years by telling lies about her to the landlord. The patient is married and is retired from a job that she held for 25 years.	A rare condition characterized by a nonbizarre, fixed delusional system (often paranoid); more common in patients older than 40 years of age, immigrants, and the hearing impaired	Content of delusions is unlikely, but not bizarre; other thought disorders are rarely present; delusional thinking is circumscribed, not affecting other areas of the patient's life
Shared psychotic disorder (folie à deux)	A 19-year-old woman whose psychotic mother believes that the police are planning to arrest her now begins to believe the same thing. This belief disappears when her mother moves out of state.	Development of delusional symptoms in a person in a close relationship with another person (usually a spouse or other family member) who has similar delusional symptoms (the inducer); more common in women and people from lower socioeconomic groups	The delusions of the patient are similar in content to those of the inducer

Table 12-2.
Treatment and Prognosis of Other Psychotic Disorders

Disorder	Treatment	Prognosis
Brief psychotic disorder	Short hospital stay, structure and support, antipsychotic medication and/or benzodiazepines, reassurance and supportive psychotherapy for dealing with the stressful precipitating event (if present)	50%–80% of patients recover completely; 20%–50% of patients ultimately may be diagnosed with schizophrenia or a mood disorder
Schizophreniform disorder	Hospitalization, antipsychotics, and supportive psychotherapy to deal with the experience of having had a psychotic episode	33% of patients recover completely; 66% progress to schizoaffective disorder or schizophrenia
Schizoaffective disorder	Hospitalization; antidepressants, antimanics, or electroconvulsive therapy; antipsychotic agents are used for psychotic episodes or may be the primary treatment if mood stabilizers are not helpful	Better than for schizophrenia, worse than for mood disorder; chronic and lifelong
Delusional disorder	Psychotherapy to gain the patient's trust, trial of pimozide (Orap), particularly for somatic delusions, or haloperidol (Haldol), although antipsychotics are often not effective	On long-term follow-up, 50% recover, 30% remain the same, and 20% show decreased symptoms; younger age at onset, sudden onset, and presence of a precipitant are associated with a good prognosis
Shared psychotic disorder (folie à deux)	Remove the patient from the influence of the inducer; social support, psychotherapy, and antipsychotic medication	10%–40% of cases resolve with separation from the inducer (such separation may be impractical if the inducer is a family member)

13

Mood Disorders

I. OVERVIEW

A. The mood, or affective, disorders are characterized by a primary disturbance in mood, causing subjective distress and occupational or social problems.

B. The DSM-IV-TR includes the following categories of mood disorders:

1. Major depressive disorder

2. Bipolar I disorder

3. Bipolar II disorder

4. Dysthymic disorder

5. Cyclothymic disorder

6. Mood disorder due to a general medical condition (see II-C below)

7. Substance induced mood disorder

C. Table 13-1 shows the lifetime prevalence, age of onset, duration of symptoms required for diagnosis, and prognosis of the first five of these mood disorders.

D. Etiology

1. The biologic causes of mood disorders include **altered neurotransmitter activity,** primarily decreased availability of serotonin and norepinephrine, and abnormalities of the limbic-hypothalamic-pituitary-adrenal axis.

2. The psychosocial etiology of depression includes loss of a parent in childhood, **social loss** during adult life (e.g., loss of a spouse), low self-esteem, loss of hope, and negative interpretation of life events (e.g., taking a genuine compliment as insincere and undeserved).

II. MAJOR DEPRESSIVE DISORDER

A. Characteristics

1. *(PATIENT SNAPSHOT)* A 40-year-old man tells his physician that he has little interest in activities he formerly enjoyed. He has lost 11 pounds, reports that he wakes up 2 hours before his alarm goes off and cannot fall back to sleep. He states "my family would be better off without me." He says that although he feels tired and "out of sorts" most of the time, he feels somewhat better in the evening than in the morning (diurnal variation in symptoms).

2. Major depressive disorder is characterized by episodes of severely depressed mood, which involve loss of pleasure and interest in most of a person's usual activities.

Table 13-1.

Lifetime Prevalence, Age of Onset, Duration of Symptoms, and Prognosis of Mood Disorders

Disorder	Lifetime Prevalence	Age of Onset	Duration of Symptoms Required for Diagnosis	Prognosis
Major depressive disorder	5%–12% for men, 10%–20% for women	Mean age of onset 40 years	At least 2 weeks	Generally, 5 or 6 depressive episodes over a 20-year period; frequency and length of episodes increase with age; approximately 75% of patients can be treated successfully; approximately 15% of patients eventually commit suicide
Bipolar disorder	1% for bipolar I, no sex difference; 0.5% for bipolar II, may be more common in women	First manic episode usually occurs before 30 years of age	Manic symptoms must last at least 1 week	Worse prognosis than major depressive disorder; interval between manic episodes (generally 6–9 months) decreases as the illness progresses
Dysthymic disorder	6%; 2–3 times more common in women	50% of patients have symptoms before 25 years of age (early-onset type)	At least 2 years	20% of patients eventually have major depressive disorder; 20% eventually have bipolar disorder (I or II); at least 25% retain depressive symptoms throughout life
Cyclothymic disorder	< 1%; occurs equally in men and women	Most common age of onset 15–25 years	At least 2 years	Chronic and lifelong; 33% eventually are diagnosed with bipolar disorder

3. As many as 50% of depressed patients seem unaware of or deny depression (**"masked depression"**), even though they have symptoms (often vague and somatic).

4. Major depressive disorder is about twice as common in women as in men.

5. The patient's mood and functioning usually return to normal between episodes.

B. Related symptoms in depressed patients

1. **Psychotic symptoms** can occur (depression with psychotic features), although fixed delusions or hallucinations are uncommon.

2. **Somatic symptoms** are common and range from mild hypochondriasis to somatic delusions (e.g., "I feel like my insides are rotting.").

3. A depressive episode has **melancholic features** if the patient has a loss of pleasure

in all or almost all activities (anhedonia) and cannot respond to pleasurable stimuli. In addition, the patient shows typical melancholic or "vegetative" signs summarized in the mnemonic SIG:E CAPS (Table 13-2).

4. Seasonal affective disorder (SAD) is a subtype of major depressive disorder associated with the winter season and short days. Many SAD patients respond to full-spectrum light exposure.

C. Differential diagnosis: medical conditions associated with depressive symptoms

1. Cancer, particularly pancreatic and other abdominal tumors

2. Viral illness [e.g., pneumonia, influenza, acquired immune deficiency syndrome (AIDS)]

3. Endocrine abnormalities, particularly thyroid dysfunction

4. Neurologic illness [e.g., Parkinson disease, multiple sclerosis, stroke (particularly left frontal)]

5. Nutritional deficiency

6. Renal or cardiopulmonary disease

7. Prescription drugs (e.g., reserpine, steroids, propranolol, methyldopa)

D. Differential diagnosis: psychiatric conditions associated with depression

1. Schizophrenia, particularly after an acute psychotic episode (see Chapter 12)

2. Anxiety disorders (see Chapter 14)

3. Drug and alcohol abuse (particularly sedatives) and withdrawal (particularly stimulants) (see Chapter 10)

4. Somatoform disorders (see Chapter 15)

E. Pharmacologic treatment

1. Antidepressants

a. Heterocyclic (tricyclic and tetracyclic) antidepressants, selective serotonin reuptake inhibitors (SSRIs), monoamine oxidase inhibitors (MAOIs), and

Table 13-2.
The Melancholic ("Vegetative") Signs of Depression: SIG:E CAPS ("Take energy capsules")

Mnemonic	Sign	Comments
S	Sleep	Insomnia and early morning awakening are common
I	Interest	Involvement in usual activities and motivation are decreased
G	Guilt	Many patients feel excessive self-blame
E	Energy	Loss of vigor is common (e.g., hard to get through routine tasks)
C	Concentration	Cognitive problems (e.g., difficulty paying attention and memory disturbances are common)
A	Appetite	Decreased desire for food and sex is common
P	Psychomotor activity	Decreased physical activity (psychomotor retardation) is common, particularly in the elderly; less often, increased physical activity (psychomotor agitation) occurs
S	Suicidal ideation	Thoughts of self-destruction are present in many patients

other antidepressants are used to treat depression (see Chapter 25). Each type of agent has advantages and disadvantages (Table 13-3).

   b. Although heterocyclics were once the mainstay of treatment, SSRIs (e.g., fluoxetine) are now used as first-line drugs.

2. Efficacy, latency of action, and combination treatments

   a. All antidepressants take at least **3–6 weeks to work.**

   b. All antidepressants **have similar efficacy.**

   c. Combinations of heterocyclic antidepressant agents and MAOIs may be used with extreme caution. Lithium or thyroid hormone (T_3) may be used to augment the efficacy of antidepressants.

   d. Patients who have depression with psychotic features may be treated with a combination of antipsychotics and antidepressants.

   e. Stimulants such as methylphenidate or dextroamphetamine may be useful to improve mood in certain patients (e.g, the terminally ill) or in individuals with refractory depression. Advantages include rapid action (i.e., no 3–6 week wait). Disadvantages include the addiction potential of stimulants and restrictions placed on their use by state licensing boards.

F. Electroconvulsive therapy (ECT)

   1. ECT is a safe and effective treatment for certain depressed patients.

   2. **ECT works quickly** and may have fewer side effects than prolonged treatment with antidepressants (Table 13-4). For this reason, it may be useful in pregnant women or elderly patients who cannot tolerate antidepressant medication side-effects.

G. Psychological treatments

   1. Psychological treatment for depression includes psychoanalytic, interpersonal, family, behavioral, and cognitive therapy (see Chapters 26, 27, and 28).

   2. Psychological treatment in conjunction with medication is more effective than either type of treatment alone.

Table 13-3.

Advantages and Disadvantages of Pharmacologic Treatments for Depression

Treatment	Advantages	Disadvantages
Heterocyclic antidepressants	No agitation or gastrointestinal upset	Sedation, anticholinergic effects, cardiovascular effects (e.g., orthostatic hypotension), weight gain; dangerous in overdose
Selective serotonin reuptake inhibitors (SSRIs)	Fewer anticholinergic and cardiovascular effects, less sedating, less weight gain (initially, minor weight loss may occur); safer in overdose	Activation and insomnia (particularly with fluoxetine); sexual problems, particularly delayed orgasm; nausea, diarrhea, other gastrointestinal upset
Monoamine oxidase inhibitors (MAOIs)	Useful for depression that does not respond to other agents, useful for "atypical" depression (e.g., mixed symptoms of anxiety and depression)	Hypertensive crisis ("cheese effect") with the ingestion of tyramine-rich foods (e.g., beer, wine, broad beans, aged cheese, beef or chicken liver, orange pulp, smoked or pickled meats or fish) or sympathomimetic drugs, dangerous in overdose

Table 13-4.
Electroconvulsive Therapy (ECT)

Description	Induction of a generalized seizure lasting 25–60 seconds by passing a current of electricity across the brain; can be unilateral (two electrodes placed on the nondominant hemisphere, one on the frontotemporal area and the other in the parietal area), bifrontal (one electrode placed above the end of each eyebrow), or bilateral (one electrode placed on each temple); fewer side effects, but less efficacy with unilateral and bifrontal than with bilateral ECT
Major indication	Major depressive disorder that is refractory to antidepressants; improvement may be seen after one treatment
Other major use	Serious depressive symptoms from any cause, particularly when rapid resolution of depressive symptoms is imperative because of suicide risk
Major side effect	Amnesia (usually retrograde), which usually remits within 6 months
How administered	After premedication (atropine) followed by general anesthesia [sodium methohexital (Brevital)] and a muscle relaxant [succinylcholine (Anectine)] given before seizure induction
Optimal number of treatments	Eight treatments over a 2- to 3-week period
Major contraindication	Increased intracranial pressure or recent (within 2 weeks) myocardial infarction
Maintenance of improvement	Antidepressant medication or outpatient electroconvulsive therapy administered once or twice monthly

H. Course

1. Untreated, an episode of depression lasts about 6–12 months and is usually **self-limiting.**

2. Only about 25% of patients with depression seek treatment.

3. Patients with severe depression often do not have energy to commit suicide. As energy returns in response to treatment, the **risk of suicide** increases.

4. Major reasons for hospitalizing a depressed patient

   a. High suicide risk (Table 13-5)
   b. Has a ready means for suicide (e.g., has a gun)
   c. Has a plan for suicide (e.g., has chosen a time)
   d. Concomitant use of alcohol or other substance of abuse
   e. Has psychotic symptoms

III. BIPOLAR DISORDER

A. Characteristics

1. Manic episode: A 28-year-old man is taken to the emergency room by police because he tried to enter a federal building to "talk to the President" about conducting a worldwide telethon to cure AIDS (grandiosity). When police prevent him from entering the building, he becomes irritable and hostile and resists the officers' attempts to restrain him (assaultive).

2. Bipolar I disorder includes episodes of both mania (very elevated mood) and major depression.

Table 13-5.
Risk Factors for Suicide

Factor	Decreased Risk	Increased Risk
TOP FIVE RISK FACTORS (IN DESCENDING ORDER)		
1) History	No previous suicidal behavior	Serious prior suicide attempt
2) Age	Younger	Older
3) Substance use	Little or no substance use	Substance abuse or dependence
4) Behavior	Not impulsive or violent	History of rage and violent behavior
5) Gender	Female	Male
OTHER RISK FACTORS		
Race	African-American	White
Social status	Married	Socially isolated
Family history	No family history of suicide	Parent or close relative committed suicide
Religion	Catholic or Muslim	Jewish or Protestant
Psychotic symptoms	No psychotic symptoms	Psychotic symptoms
Health	Good health	Chronic illness
Occupation	Non-professional	Professional
Economic conditions	Strong economy	Economic recession or depression
Employment	Job satisfaction	Low job satisfaction

3. Bipolar II disorder includes episodes of both hypomania (elevated mood, but not as severe as in mania) and major depression.

4. The depressed phase of bipolar disorder resembles depression in major depressive disorder, but the first episode may differ. Conditions associated with a first episode of depression that predict bipolar disorder include:

   a. Depression characterized by psychotic symptoms or psychomotor retardation
   b. Mania or hypomania after antidepressant drug therapy
   c. Postpartum depression

5. Untreated manic episodes last approximately 3 months. There is no unipolar manic disorder because depressive symptoms eventually occur. Therefore, one episode of mania or hypomania defines bipolar disorder.

B. Differential diagnosis

   1. Schizophrenia (Chapter 11)

   2. Schizoaffective disorder (Chapter 12)

   3. Substance abuse (Chapter 10)

   4. Delirium (Chapter 9)

   5. Cyclothymic disorder (see below)

   6. Endocrine abnormalities, particularly thyroid dysfunction

C. Occurrence

   1. Risk of bipolar disorder:

      a. 75% for monozygotic twins of patients with bipolar disorder
      b. 60% for people with two parents who have bipolar disorder
      c. 20% for first-degree relatives (i.e., child, sibling) of patients with bipolar disorder
      d. 1% for the general population

2. **No ethnic differences are seen,** but in poor African-American and Hispanic patients, mood disorders (particularly bipolar disorder) are often misdiagnosed as schizophrenia.

D. Treatment (and see Chapter 19)

1. The drug of choice for the long-term treatment of mania is **lithium;** the drug of choice for the emergency room treatment of a manic episode is an antipsychotic like haloperidol (Haldol).

2. Lithium is used also to **control aggressive behavior** and enhance the activity of tricyclic antidepressants.

3. Anticonvulsants, such as **carbamazepine** (Tegretol) and **valproic acid** (Depakene), or **divalproex** (Depakote), are also used to treat bipolar disorder, particularly the rapid cycling type (i.e., more than four episodes annually) and mixed episodes (mixed manic and depressive features).

    a. Newer anticonvulsants that have mood-stabilizing effects include lamotrigine (Lamictal), gabapentin (Neurontin), topiramate (Topamax), and tiagabine (Gabatril).

    b. Anticonvulsants are also used to treat bipolar symptoms associated with cognitive disorders.

IV. DYSTHYMIC AND CYCLOTHYMIC DISORDERS

A. Characteristics

1. Dysthymic disorder: A 26-year-old woman has felt "low" since her college graduation 4 years ago. Her family members say that she never seems really happy. She resists their suggestions that she seek psychotherapy.

2. Dysthymic disorder involves mild or moderate depression most of the time, with **no discrete episodes.**

3. Cyclothymic disorder: A 30-year-old woman has seemed full of energy and optimism for no obvious reason (an "up," or hypomanic, period) for the last 4 months. Previously, she was described by friends and family as "down in the dumps."

4. Cyclothymic disorder involves episodes of both hypomania and mild or moderate depression.

5. The diagnosis of dysthymic disorder or cyclothymic disorder is not made until the patient has had **symptoms for at least 2 years.**

B. Differential diagnosis

1. The most common differential diagnosis of dysthymic disorder is bereavement or adjustment disorder with depressed mood. In contrast to dysthymic disorder, in bereavement (Chapter 6) or adjustment disorder (Chapter 20) a clearly identifiable life stress precipitates the depressive symptoms, which remit over time.

2. Substance abuse, particularly abuse of central nervous system (CNS) depressants, may resemble dysthymia; patients taking CNS stimulants may look hypomanic (Chapter 10).

3. Major depressive disorder is episodic and severe, and results in profoundly impaired social and occupational functioning. Dysthymic disorder is nonepisodic, chronic, less severe, results in mild, moderate, or severe impairment in functioning, and is never associated with psychosis.

4. In some patients with major depressive disorder, the residual phase is characterized by dysthymic disorder (**"double depression"**).

C. **Etiology.** Chronic medical illness in childhood and loss of a close relative are implicated in the etiology of dysthymic disorder.

D. Treatment

1. The most effective psychological treatments for dysthymic disorder are cognitive therapy (see Chapter 27) and insight-oriented psychotherapy (see Chapter 26).

2. Although formerly considered ineffective, antidepressants are now commonly used to treat dysthymic disorder.

3. MAOIs and SSRIs are more effective than heterocyclic agents in dysthymic patients with significant anxiety.

4. Antimanic agents in doses similar to those used to treat bipolar disorder are the primary treatment for cyclothymic disorder.

14

Anxiety Disorders

I. OVERVIEW

A. General characteristics

1. Anxiety disorders are characterized by subjective and physical manifestations of **fear.**

2. An anxious person experiences apprehension, but in contrast to the experience of actual fear, the source of the danger is not known, not recognized, or inadequate to account for the symptoms.

3. The **physiologic manifestations** of anxiety are similar to those of fear, including shakiness, palpitations (i.e., subjective experience of tachycardia), perioral loss of sensation, sweating, dizziness, mydriasis (pupil dilation), syncope, tingling in the extremities, gastrointestinal disturbances, and urinary urgency and frequency.

B. Etiology

1. Biologic, psychosocial, and genetic factors may contribute to the development of the anxiety disorders.

2. Neurotransmitters involved include γ-aminobutyric acid (GABA; decreased activity), serotonin (decreased activity), and norepinephrine (increased activity).

3. Medical conditions associated with the symptoms of anxiety include excessive caffeine intake, substance abuse, vitamin B_{12} deficiency, hyperthyroidism, hypoglycemia, cardiac arrhythmias, mitral valve prolapse, and pheochromocytoma (an adrenal medullary tumor).

C. Classification

1. The five major DSM-IV-TR classifications of anxiety disorders are:

   a. Panic disorder with or without agoraphobia
   b. Phobias (specific and social)
   c. Obsessive-compulsive disorder (OCD)
   d. Generalized anxiety disorder (GAD)
   e. Posttraumatic stress disorder (PTSD) and acute stress disorder (ASD)

2. Other classifications of anxiety disorders include:

   a. Anxiety disorder due to a general medical condition
   b. Substance-induced anxiety disorder

3. Table 14-1 shows the differential diagnosis of anxiety disorders.

4. Table 14-2 describes the treatment of anxiety disorders.

Table 14-1.
Differential Diagnosis of Anxiety Disorders

Classification	Psychological Differential Diagnosis	Physical Differential Diagnosis
Panic disorder with or without agoraphobia	Social or specific phobia, generalized anxiety disorder, depression, schizophrenia (prodrome), malingering, hypochondriasis, factitious disorder	Myocardial infarction (because shortness of breath, chest discomfort, tachycardia, and sweating occur in both), cardiac arrhythmias, mitral valve prolapse, hyperthyroidism, pheochromocytoma, hyperparathyroidism, stimulant use, central nervous system depressant (sedative) withdrawal
Specific phobia	Obsessive-compulsive disorder, hypochondriasis, paranoid personality disorder, panic disorder, delusional disorder, anorexia nervosa, bulimia nervosa	. . .
Social phobia	Normal shyness, schizoid personality disorder, avoidant personality disorder, panic disorder, major depressive disorder	. . .
Obsessive-compulsive disorder	Schizophrenia, obsessive-compulsive personality disorder	Tourette disorder, temporal lobe epilepsy
Generalized anxiety disorder	Other anxiety disorders, particularly panic disorder	Hyperthyroidism, excessive caffeine intake, stimulant use, sedative withdrawal
Posttraumatic stress disorder	Generalized anxiety disorder, substance abuse, borderline personality disorder, factitious disorder, malingering; the most important distinguishing factor between posttraumatic stress disorder and these disorders is the presence of a catastrophic traumatic event in the patient's history	Brain injury caused by a traumatic event

II. PANIC DISORDER (WITH OR WITHOUT AGORAPHOBIA)

A. Characteristics

1. A 22-year-old female medical student comes to the emergency room with tachycardia, sweating, and dyspnea, certain that she is having a heart attack. The symptoms started suddenly when she was in a shopping mall. Other than an elevated pulse rate, the findings of physical examination are normal.

2. Panic disorder consists of **panic attacks,** defined as episodic periods of anxiety symptoms that have a sudden onset and increase in intensity over a period of approximately 10 minutes.

3. Panic attacks occur approximately **twice weekly** and last approximately **30 minutes.** Between attacks, the patient fears having another attack (anticipatory anxiety).

4. Panic disorder with **agoraphobia** consists of panic attacks that are triggered by

Table 14-2.
Treatment of Anxiety Disorders

Classification	Treatment (in descending order of utility for each classification)	
	Pharmacologic treatment	**Psychologic treatment**
Panic disorder with or without agoraphobia	For acute treatment or anticipatory anxiety: Benzodiazepines, particularly alprazolam (Xanax); pharmacologic treatment is continued for 8–12 months, with gradual withdrawal; some patients do well with much lower initial doses For maintenance: Selective serotonin reuptake inhibitors (SSRIs), tricyclics, monoamine oxidase inhibitors (MAOIs)	Systematic desensitization and cognitive therapy are useful adjuncts to pharmacotherapy
Specific phobia	No effective pharmacologic treatment; short-term benzodiazepines and β-blockers to control autonomic symptoms may help during desensitization.	Systematic desensitization with reciprocal inhibition is most effective (see Chapter 27); hypnosis, family therapy, and psychotherapy are also useful
Social phobia	Antidepressants, primarily MAOIs; β-blockers to control autonomic symptoms, particularly for performance or test anxiety	Assertiveness training and group therapy are useful
Obsessive-compulsive disorder	SSRIs, the strongly serotonergic tricyclic antidepressant clomipramine (Anafranil); all must be titrated slowly up to the effective dose	The most useful psychological treatments are behavior therapy (e.g., flooding, implosion; see Chapter 27); supportive psychotherapy may also be useful (see Chapter 26)
Generalized anxiety disorder	Benzodiazepines, particularly those that have an intermediate length of action, because they work rapidly, last for a reasonably long time, and have less addiction potential than short-acting agents; buspirone (BuSpar) is most useful for patients who have never been treated with or who cannot use benzodiazepines (although it takes 2–3 weeks to work); antidepressants such as venlafaxine (Effexor) and doxepin (Adapin or Sinequan); β-blockers are used primarily for autonomic symptoms	Because benzodiazepines carry a high risk of dependence and addiction, they are used primarily for acute exacerbations of symptoms (weeks to months); cognitive therapy and behavioral therapy are more useful for chronic symptoms
Posttraumatic stress disorder	No good pharmacologic treatment, although the following agents have been tried with some success: antidepressants, such as sertraline (Zoloft); anticonvulsants, particularly for flashbacks and nightmares; β-blockers to control autonomic symptoms	Psychological treatment, including psychotherapy and support groups (e.g., victim survivor groups); group therapy must be initiated as soon as possible after the traumatic event

exposure to an open space (e.g., when the patient goes outside of his home alone) or by a situation in which the patient cannot escape or obtain help.

B. Diagnosis

   1. For diagnostic purposes, a panic attack can be induced in a patient with panic disorder by **IV administration of sodium lactate** in a physician's office. Hyperventilation or inhalation of CO_2 (breathing into and out of a paper bag) also can provoke a panic attack.

   2. Although panic disorder is associated with mitral valve prolapse, no causal relation is known.

   3. Depression is present in approximately 50% of patients with panic disorder.

C. Occurrence

   1. The mean age of **onset of panic disorder is 25 years.**

   2. Panic disorder is **more common in women.**

   3. Panic disorder has a lifetime prevalence of 1.5–3.5%.

   4. **Genetic factors** are involved; first-degree relatives (i.e., sibling, child) have a four to seven times greater chance of having panic disorder.

   5. Panic disorder may occur soon after divorce or marital separation.

   6. Panic disorder with agoraphobia is associated with **separation anxiety disorder** of childhood (see Chapter 5).

D. Prognosis

   1. Panic disorder has a chronic course, with many recurrent episodes.

   2. As many as 90% of patients experience a relapse when medication is discontinued.

III. PHOBIAS

A. Characteristics

   1. *(PATIENT SNAPSHOT)* **Specific phobia:** A 32-year-old woman who is terrified of dogs refuses to leave her house to go to work because she may see a dog on the street.

   2. **Specific phobia** is an irrational fear of certain situations or objects (e.g., animals, heights, needles). The patient avoids the feared situation or object.

   3. *(PATIENT SNAPSHOT)* **Social phobia:** A 29-year-old man is uncomfortable because he must take a client to dinner in a restaurant. Although he knows the client well, he is so afraid that he will make a mess while eating and embarrass himself that he says he is not hungry and sips from a glass of water instead.

   4. **Social phobia** is an exaggerated fear of social or environmental situations (e.g., public speaking, eating in public, using public restrooms). The patient avoids the feared situation.

B. Occurrence

   1. Specific phobia has a lifetime prevalence of 7%–11% in the population.

   2. Social phobia has a lifetime prevalence of 3%–13% of the population.

C. **Prognosis.** Patients with specific or social phobias often have **secondary morbidity** (e.g., employment impairment, school dropout, failure to marry).

IV. OBSESSIVE-COMPULSIVE DISORDER (OCD)

A. Characteristics

1. Before she can go to sleep at night, a 25-year-old woman counts the tiles on the ceiling at least five times. She has had a few minor car accidents because she is distracted by counting traffic lights.

2. Patients with OCD experience recurring intrusive feelings, thoughts, and images **(obsessions)** which cause anxiety that is relieved in part by performing repetitive actions **(compulsions).**

3. The most common obsessions and compulsions include **contamination** (e.g., cleansing after touching common objects), **checking** (e.g., "Have I hit someone with my car?"), **counting,** and **putting things in order.**

4. Patients usually realize that these thoughts and behaviors are irrational (symptoms are ego-dystonic) and want to eliminate them (i.e., **they have insight).**

B. Etiology

1. Electroencephalographic (EEG) abnormalities in sleep studies [e.g., decreased rapid eye movement (REM) latency] and neuroendocrine abnormalities are similar to those seen in patients with depression.

2. Based on the effectiveness of selective serotonin reuptake inhibitors (SSRIs) and the strongly serotonergic tricyclic antidepressant clomipramine (Anafranil) in treating OCD, it appears that **serotonin** is a closely associated neurotransmitter.

3. Psychosocial factors may also be involved; symptoms of OCD often first appear after a stressful life experience.

4. Genetic factors also play a role: the concordance rate is increased in first-degree relatives of patients with OCD and is higher in monozygotic than in dizygotic twins.

5. OCD is associated with other anxiety disorders, major depressive disorder, obsessive-compulsive personality disorder, eating disorders, and Tourette disorder.

C. Occurrence

1. OCD usually starts in early adulthood, but may begin in childhood.

2. OCD occurs in 2–3% of the population.

3. OCD is seen equally in men and women.

D. Prognosis. In one-third of patients, symptoms improve significantly with treatment. In one-half, symptoms improve moderately. In the rest, symptoms do not improve or progressive deterioration in functioning occurs.

V. GENERALIZED ANXIETY DISORDER (GAD)

A. Characteristics

1. A 40-year-old woman says that she frequently experiences "palpitations," shortness of breath, and chronic indigestion. She says that for as long as she can remember, she has felt "tense and nervous."

2. Patients with GAD have persistent symptoms of anxiety, including hyperarousal, that **last at least 6 months.**

3. The symptoms of anxiety in GAD are unrelated to a specific person or situation **("free-floating" anxiety).**

4. GAD is closely associated with major depressive disorder and dysthymic disorder.

B. Occurrence

  1. The lifetime prevalence of GAD is about 5%.

  2. GAD is slightly more common in women (55%–60%) than in men (40%–45%).

  3. In 50% of patients, onset occurs during childhood or adolescence.

C. Prognosis. Approximately one-half of patients with GAD have **chronic symptoms** which wax and wane and require treatment indefinitely. The remaining patients become asymptomatic within a few years. A major complication of long-term treatment is addiction to benzodiazepine antianxiety agents.

VI. POSTTRAUMATIC STRESS DISORDER (PTSD)

A. Characteristics

  1. A 35-year-old woman who was raped 5 years ago has recurrent vivid memories of the rape accompanied by intense anxiety. These memories frequently intrude during her daily activities, and nightmares about the event often wake her. Her symptoms intensified when a coworker was raped 2 months ago.

  2. PTSD occurs when a **catastrophic event** (usually life-threatening or potentially fatal, e.g., war, terrorist attack like 9/11, earthquake, serious accident or robbery) affects the patient or a close friend or relative.

  3. The patient experiences symptoms of both **hyperarousal** and **withdrawal.**

    a. Symptoms of hyperarousal include anxiety, recurrent nightmares, intrusive memories of the event (flashbacks), increased startle response, and hypervigilance.
    b. Symptoms of withdrawal include numbing of affective response, survivor's guilt, dissociation, and social withdrawal.

  4. For a diagnosis of PTSD, **symptoms must last for more than 1 month;** in chronic PTSD, symptoms can last for years. Symptoms that last between 2 days and 4 weeks following a catastrophic event are diagnosed as **acute stress disorder** (ASD) rather than PTSD.

  5. Psychological symptoms occurring after a serious or even catastrophic (but not usually life-threatening) life event (e.g., bankruptcy, divorce) indicate adjustment disorder (see Chapter 20).

B. Occurrence. The lifetime prevalence of PTSD is about 8% in the general population and up to half of people who are at particular risk (e.g., earthquake survivors, combat veterans).

C. Prognosis. One-half of patients with PTSD recover completely within 3 months. Many others have symptoms for a year or longer.

15

Somatoform Disorders, Factitious Disorder, and Malingering

I. SOMATOFORM DISORDERS

A. Characteristics

1. Somatoform disorders are characterized by **physical symptoms without a sufficient organic cause.** A person who has a somatoform disorder is not faking and not delusional, but truly believes that he or she has a physical problem.

2. The five major DSM-IV-TR classifications of somatoform disorders (Tables 15-1 and 15-2) are:

    a. Somatization disorder
    b. Conversion disorder
    c. Hypochondriasis
    d. Body dysmorphic disorder
    e. Pain disorder
    f. Somatoform disorder not otherwise specified (NOS)

B. Differential diagnosis

1. The most important differential diagnosis of the somatoform disorders is unidentified organic disease.

2. Physical illnesses most likely to be misdiagnosed as somatoform disorders are:

    a. Early-stage connective tissue disorders (e.g., systemic lupus erythematosus [SLE], rheumatoid arthritis)

    b. Central nervous system (CNS) disorders (e.g., brain tumor, multiple sclerosis, epilepsy)

    c. Endocrine and metabolic disorders (e.g., hypoglycemia, thyroid dysfunction, porphyria)

3. Factitious disorder and malingering (faking illness) must be excluded.

4. Psychotic disorders with somatic delusions must also be excluded.

C. Occurrence

1. Most somatoform disorders are more common in women, although hypochondriasis occurs equally in men and women.

2. Fifty percent of patients with a somatoform disorder also have another mental disorder (most commonly depression or anxiety).

Table 15-1.
Characteristics of Somatoform Disorders

Disorder		Patient Snapshot	Characteristics
Somatization disorder		A 45-year-old woman has a 20-year history of vague and chronic physical complaints. She says that she has always been sick but that her doctors never seem to identify the problem and cannot help her.	A history of multiple somatic complaints over many years, including: • 4 pain symptoms (e.g., headache) • 2 gastrointestinal symptoms (e.g., nausea) • 1 sexual symptom (e.g., menstrual irregularities) • 1 pseudoneurologic symptom (e.g., paralysis)
Conversion disorder		A 28-year-old woman experiences a sudden loss of vision, but appears unconcerned ("la belle indifference"). She reports that just before the onset of her blindness, she saw her child dart out into the street.	Abrupt, dramatic loss of motor or sensory function (e.g., hearing, vision), often with an obvious or symbolic significance; the most common motor symptoms are paralysis (shifting to different areas of the body; pathologic reflexes are absent), seizures (often bizarre), and globus hystericus (i.e., lump in the throat); the most common sensory presentations are paresthesias (abnormal sensations), anesthesias [often inconsistent with anatomic innervation (e.g., "stocking and glove" distribution)], and visual problems (e.g., blindness, tunnel vision); evoked potentials are normal (see Chapter 3)
Hypochondriasis		A 41-year-old man says that he has been "ill" for most of his life. He has seen many doctors ("doctor shopping"), but is angry with most of them because they ultimately referred him to mental health clinicians. He now fears that he has stomach cancer because his stomach makes noises after he eats. Many of his previous "illnesses" also seem to be amplified responses to normal physical sensations.	Exaggerated concern with health and illness over at least a 6-month period that continues despite medical evaluation and reassurance by a physician.

(continued)

Table 15-1.—*Continued*
Characteristics of Somatoform Disorders

Disorder		Patient Snapshot	Characteristics
Body dysmorphic disorder		A 28-year-old woman seeks blepharoplasty for her "sagging" eyelids. She rarely goes out in the daytime because she believes that this characteristic makes her look "like an old lady." On physical examination, her eyelids appear completely normal.	Excessive focus on a minor or imagined physical defect (usually of the face or head)
Pain disorder		A 40-year-old man who had a minor knee injury playing ball 11 months ago continues to complain of severe knee pain, although there is little or no evidence of any abnormality.	Protracted, intense discomfort not explained adequately by physical causes; can be acute (lasting < 6 months) or chronic (lasting > 6 months) and often coexists with a medical condition
Somatoform disorder not otherwise specified		A 40-year-old woman reports that she often feels nauseated. This symptom causes her to lose time from work. Physical and laboratory examinations are normal.	Persistent physical symptoms (not feigned) that do not meet the full criteria for another somatoform disorder. Most common are fatigue, gastrointestinal or genitourinary complaints, and loss of appetite.

D. Etiology

   1. Genetic factors are associated with most somatoform disorders.

   2. Although the patient is not consciously aware of it, primary or secondary gain is often a result of the symptoms.

   a. The patient unconsciously expresses an unacceptable feeling as a physical symptom so that he does not have to deal with the feeling **(primary gain).**

   b. The physical symptom serves a useful purpose, such as getting attention from others or avoiding responsibility **(secondary gain).**

E. Treatment

   1. Useful strategies for treatment

   a. Forming a good physician–patient relationship (e.g., scheduling regular appointments, providing reassurance)

   b. Decreasing the secondary gain associated with the symptoms

   c. Evaluating the patient's social support system and identifying and decreasing the difficulties in the patient's life that may aggravate the symptoms

   d. Maintaining a close collaboration with the patient's other treating physicians

   e. Emphasizing management (rather than cure) as the goal of treatment

   2. Pharmacologic and psychological therapies

   a. Pharmacotherapy has limited usefulness unless the patient has a comorbid psychiatric illness (e.g., depression, anxiety).

Table 15-2.
Occurrence, Course, and Prognosis of Somatoform Disorders

Disorder	Occurrence	Course and Prognosis
Somatization disorder	Onset before 30 years of age; specific symptoms vary by culture	Chronic and lifelong; symptoms are increased by stressful life events
Conversion disorder	More common in psychiatrically unsophisticated patients (e.g., adolescents, young adults, patients from rural areas); comorbid with histrionic personality disorder	Symptoms often remit in < 1 month, sometimes immediately after hypnosis or sodium amobarbital interview (see Chapter 3); symptoms recur in approximately one-fourth of patients, particularly during stressful life events
Hypochondriasis	More common in middle and old age	Symptoms may last for as long as a few years; these periods alternate with periods when few symptoms are present; as many as 50% of patients improve over the course of their lives
Body dysmorphic disorder	Onset usually in the late teens	Level of concern varies over time; plastic surgery or other medical treatment must be used cautiously because it rarely relieves the symptoms
Pain disorder	Onset usually in the thirties and forties	Can be disabling, particularly if there is a significant physiological component to the patient's symptoms; patient may become dependent on pain medication; antidepressants with serotonergic action (e.g., selective serotonin reuptake inhibitors) may be useful

    b. Individual and group psychotherapy, hypnosis, behavioral and relaxation therapy can be useful.

    c. Either pharmacologic or psychological treatment can control the disorder, but symptoms often return.

II. FACTITIOUS DISORDER (MUNCHAUSEN SYNDROME) AND FACTITIOUS DISORDER BY PROXY

  A. Characteristics

    1. Factitious disorder by proxy: A 34-year-old woman takes her 8-year-old daughter to a physician's office. She says that the child often experiences bouts of severe dyspnea and abdominal pain. The child's medical record shows many office visits and four abdominal surgical procedures that resulted in a "grid abdomen" due to crossed surgical scarring, although no abnormalities were ever found. When she is confronted with the doctor's suspicion that illness in the child is being faked by the mother, the mother angrily grabs the child and immediately leaves the office.

    2. In contrast to patients with somatoform disorders (who really believe that they are ill), patients with factitious disorder know that they are pretending to have a mental or physical illness or actually inducing physical illness to obtain medical attention. In factitious disorder by proxy, an adult, usually a parent, feigns or induces illness in a child to obtain medical attention.

3. Patients often have worked in the medical field (e.g., nurses, technicians) and know how to simulate an illness.

4. The most commonly feigned symptoms are abdominal pain, fever (by heating the thermometer), blood in the urine (by adding blood from a needle stick), induction of tachycardia (by drug administration), skin lesions (by injuring easily reached areas), and seizures.

5. Factitious disorder by proxy is a form of child abuse and must be reported to child welfare authorities.

B. Etiology

1. Patients often have a history of serious childhood illness that resulted in medical treatment or hospitalization. During this illness, the patient felt cared for and protected. In adulthood, the patient continues to seek medical care.

2. The patient may have a history of childhood abuse or neglect.

C. Course and prognosis

1. Because the patient is preoccupied with illness and medical care, work (or school) and social relationships may suffer.

2. The patient (or in factitious disorder by proxy, the child) may undergo unnecessary medical procedures or receive unnecessary medication with all of its complications.

III. MALINGERING

A. Characteristics

1. A 48-year-old man claims that he injured his back at work. He asserts that his injury prevents him from working and interferes with his marital relationship. He has no further sign of back problems after he receives a $50,000 worker's compensation settlement, but still does not return to work.

2. Malingering is the conscious simulation or exaggeration of physical or mental illness for financial or other obvious gain (e.g., avoiding work or incarceration).

B. Course and prognosis. In contrast to the patient with factitious disorder who seeks medical treatment, the malingering patient avoids treatment. His symptoms often improve after he obtains the desired gain.

16

Dissociative Disorders

I. OVERVIEW

A. General Characteristics

    1. Dissociative disorders are characterized by sudden but temporary **loss of memory** or **identity** or by feelings of **detachment** because of emotional factors.

    2. The four major DSM-IV-TR classifications of dissociative disorders are:

        a. Dissociative amnesia

        b. Dissociative fugue

        c. Dissociative identity disorder (multiple personality disorder)

        d. Depersonalization disorder and derealization

    3. Table 16-1 shows the occurrence, etiology, treatment, course, and prognosis of dissociative disorders.

B. Differential diagnosis

    1. The medical differential diagnosis of dissociative disorders includes substance abuse, head injury, sequelae of electroconvulsive therapy (ECT) or anesthesia, seizure disorder, delirium, and dementia.

    2. The psychological differential diagnosis of the dissociative disorders includes post-traumatic stress disorder (PTSD) and malingering.

    3. Members of some religions or cultures view altered states of perception, identity, or consciousness in the framework of particular experiences (e.g., a trance state entered into at a religious revival meeting). In these frameworks, dissociation may not be abnormal.

II. DISSOCIATIVE AMNESIA (PSYCHOGENIC AMNESIA)

A. A 20-year-old soldier cannot recall the events of a battle in which one-half of his platoon was killed.

B. Dissociative amnesia is characterized by an inability to recall important data about oneself.

III. DISSOCIATIVE FUGUE (PSYCHOGENIC FUGUE)

A. A 32-year-old secretary who formerly lived in New York has been living in Oregon and working as a cashier for more than 3 years. She has no memory of coming to Oregon or of living in New York.

Table 16-1.

Occurrence, Etiology, Treatment, Course, and Prognosis of Dissociative Disorders

Disorder	Occurrence	Etiology	Treatment	Course and Prognosis
Dissociative amnesia	Uncommon; usually affects young adults and women	Use of the defense mechanisms of repression and denial after a recent emotionally traumatic event	Hypnosis and sodium amobarbital interview (see Chapter 3) to recover the traumatic memories; long-term psychotherapy to deal with the recovered material	Amnesia after acute stress usually resolves in minutes or days; occasionally lasts for years
Dissociative fugue	Rare; associated with a history of excessive alcohol use			
Dissociative identity disorder (multiple personality disorder)	In mild form, more common than previously believed; rare in severe form; much more common in women	Early traumatic experiences, particularly abuse in childhood or adolescence; most commonly associated with incest	In some cases, insight-oriented psychotherapy with or without hypnosis, is effective in integrating the alters; antidepressants, antianxiety, antipsychotic and anticonvulsant agents may be useful	Often chronic and associated with other psychiatric symptoms (e.g., depression, anxiety)
Depersonalization disorder	Often occurs normally in transient form, particularly after acute stress	Exposure to severe psychological stress. Anxiety and depression are precipitating factors.	Antianxiety agents and selective serotonin reuptake inhibitors may be useful; psychotherapy is rarely useful	Usually begins between 15 and 30 years of age, occurs episodically, and commonly continues for many years

B. Dissociative fugue is characterized by the sudden inability to remember pertinent personal information coupled with leaving home, moving away, and taking on a different identity. The person is usually not aware that she has assumed a new identity.

IV. DISSOCIATIVE IDENTITY DISORDER (MULTIPLE PERSONALITY DISORDER)

A. A 35-year-old woman who is married and has two children usually dresses conservatively. She receives a letter containing a recent photograph of herself in a low-cut sweater and a short skirt. She does not remember the man who wrote the letter. She has no recollection of purchasing the outfit or posing for the photograph.

B. Dissociative identity disorder is characterized by at least two separate personalities, or "alters," within one individual. Patients often have five to ten alters, or more.

C. Most patients are women (although some of the alters may be male), and one personality usually rules the others.

D. Mild forms of dissociative identity disorder may resemble borderline personality disorder or schizophrenia.

E. When the patient presents in a legal or forensic setting (e.g., the person is in jail for a crime he claims he does not remember), malingering (Chapter 15) and alcohol abuse must be excluded.

V. DEPERSONALIZATION DISORDER

A. A 40-year-old man says that he feels as if he is "outside of himself" watching his life as though it were a movie. He knows that his perception is only a feeling and that he is really living his life (i.e., the patient has normal reality testing).

B. Depersonalization disorder is characterized by recurrent and persistent feelings of detachment from the self, social situation, or environment (derealization).

C. Symptoms of depersonalization and derealization often occur in patients with other psychiatric disorders, such as schizophrenia, depression, anxiety, and histrionic and borderline personality disorder.

17

Sexual and Gender Identity Disorders

I. SEXUAL DYSFUNCTIONS: OVERVIEW

A. The sexual response cycle

    1. Sexual dysfunctions involve difficulty with an aspect of the sexual response cycle without an identifiable biologic basis.

    2. Stages of the sexual response cycle (Table 17-1) include **excitement, plateau, orgasm,** and **resolution.**

B. Sexual disorder classifications in DSM-IV-TR

    1. The sexual desire disorders are **hypoactive sexual desire** and **sexual aversion** (disorders of the excitement phase).

    2. The sexual arousal disorders are **female sexual arousal disorder** and **male erectile disorder** (disorders of the excitement and plateau phases).

    3. The orgasmic disorders are **male orgasmic disorder, female orgasmic disorder,** and **premature ejaculation** (disorders of the orgasm phase).

    4. The sexual pain disorders are **dyspareunia** and **vaginismus** (not due to a general medical condition).

    5. Table 17-2 shows characteristics and patient snapshots of sexual dysfunctions.

C. Differential diagnosis

    1. Unidentified general medical condition (e.g., diabetes can cause erectile dysfunction; pelvic adhesions can cause dyspareunia)

    2. Side effects of medication (e.g., selective serotonin reuptake inhibitors can cause delayed orgasm), substance use, or substance abuse (e.g., alcohol use can cause erectile dysfunction)

    3. Alterations in the levels of the gonadal hormones (estrogen, progesterone, and testosterone), which are involved in sexual interest and expression (Table 17-3)

    4. In men with erectile disorder, the presence of morning erections, erections during masturbation, or erections during rapid eye movement (REM) sleep suggests a psychological rather than a physical cause.

D. Occurrence

    1. Most common male sexual dysfunctions

        a. Premature ejaculation

Table 17-1.
Characteristics of the Sexual Response Cycle

Stage	Men	Women	Both Men and Women
Excitement	Penile erection	Clitoral erection, labial swelling, vaginal lubrication, tenting effect (rising of the uterus in the pelvic cavity)	Increased pulse, blood pressure, and respiration; nipple erection
Plateau	Increased size and upward movement of the testes, secretion of a few drops of sperm-containing fluid (pre-ejaculate)	Contraction of the outer one-third of the vagina, forming the orgasmic platform (enlargement of the upper one-third of the vagina)	Further increase in pulse, blood pressure, and respiration; flushing of the chest and face
Orgasm	Forcible expulsion of seminal fluid	Contractions of the uterus and vagina	Contractions of the anal sphincter; further increases in pulse, blood pressure, and respiration
Resolution	Refractory, or resting, period (length varies by age and physical condition) when restimulation is not possible	Little or no refractory period	Muscle relaxation and return of the sexual and cardiovascular systems to the prestimulated state over a 10- to 15-minute period

     b. Erectile disorder in a man who has previously had erections (i.e., secondary erectile disorder)

  2. Most common female sexual dysfunctions

     a. Hypoactive sexual desire disorder
     b. Orgasmic disorder

E. Psychological etiology

  1. Current **relationship problems**

  2. Long-term psychological problems (e.g., chronic depression)

  3. Incompatible sexual technique between partners

  4. Fear and anxiety due to:

     a. Unconscious factors (e.g., guilt because of strict religious upbringing)
     b. Performance anxiety (e.g., because of previous erectile failure or alcohol use)
     c. Fear of pregnancy or commitment
     d. Fear of rejection or loss of control (especially with orgasmic disorders)

F. Treatment

  1. Sex therapy

     a. Increasingly, **primary care physicians** are treating patients with sexual problems instead of referring them to sex therapists.

Table 17-2.

DSM-IV Sexual Dysfunctions: Characteristics and Patient Snapshots

Disorder (prevalence estimate in people age 18–59)	Characteristics		Patient Snapshot
Hypoactive sexual desire (33%)	Decreased interest in sexual activity (may be normal individual variation in desire)		A 44-year-old man who has been married for 20 years says that although he still loves his wife, he no longer feels much desire to have sex with her or with anyone else.
Sexual aversion disorder (prevalence not available)	Aversion to and avoidance of sexual activity		A 23-year-old woman (who does not have lesbian interests) enjoys dating men, but dislikes all sexual activity with them, including kissing.
Female sexual arousal disorder (20%)	Inability to maintain vaginal lubrication until the sex act is completed, despite adequate physical stimulation		A 32-year-old woman reports that although she is interested in engaging in sexual interaction with her husband (whom she describes as a patient, sensitive lover), she does not become physically aroused during their sexual activity.
Male erectile disorder (commonly called "impotence") (10%)	• Lifelong or **primary** (rare): Has never had an erection sufficient for penetration • Acquired or **secondary** (common): Current inability to maintain erections despite normal erections in the past • Situational (common): Difficulty maintaining erections in some situations, but not others		A 39-year-old man (who has never before had problems with erections) begins to have difficulty achieving an erection during sexual activity with his wife. The very first time he had trouble maintaining an erection was at a beach party when he had "too much to drink." He now has erectile problems even when he does not drink.
Orgasmic disorder (male 10% and female 25%)	• **Lifelong:** No previous orgasm • **Acquired:** Current inability to achieve orgasm despite adequate genital stimulation (normal orgasms in the past)		Although she reports that she is sexually aroused, a 39-year-old woman has never reached orgasm by any means—during sexual activity with her husband, with stimulation devices, or during masturbation.
Premature ejaculation (27%)	Ejaculation before the man would like it to occur; short or absent plateau phase of the sexual response cycle; usually accompanied by anxiety		A 32-year-old man says that he usually has an orgasm and ejaculates before he achieves vaginal penetration.

(continued)

Table 17-2.—*Continued*
DSM-IV Sexual Dysfunctions: Characteristics and Patient Snapshots

Disorder (prevalence estimate in people age 18–59)	Characteristics		Patient Snapshot
Vaginismus (prevalence not available)	Painful spasm of the outer one-third of the vagina	*PATIENT SNAPSHOT*	A 27-year-old couple married for 4 years have never had sexual intercourse because the wife has vaginal muscle spasms which prevent the husband from achieving vaginal penetration even though he has a full erection. Although examination of the woman's external genitalia shows no abnormalities, a speculum cannot be readily inserted into the vagina (because of muscle contraction and pain).
Dyspareunia (male 3% and female 15%)	Persistent pain associated with sexual intercourse; can occur in men	*PATIENT SNAPSHOT*	A 24-year-old woman experiences pelvic pain when she and her boyfriend attempt to have sexual intercourse. No abnormalities are found during pelvic examination.

b. Patients who have serious relationship problems or a history of sexual abuse or rape may benefit from marital counseling and dual sex therapy (a male and a female therapist see the couple together; see Chapter 28).

2. Behavioral therapy and relaxation techniques, including hypnosis (see Chapter

Table 17-3.
Gonadal Hormones and Human Sexuality

Hormone	Comments
Estrogen	Involved only minimally in sexual response in women; therefore, menopause (cessation of ovarian estrogen production) and aging do not cause decreased sex drive, but often cause peripheral problems (e.g., vaginal dryness, atrophy) that can be reversed with estrogen replacement therapy; used in men to treat prostate cancer because it decreases androgen secretion. However, estrogen may reduce sexual interest and behavior in men.
Progesterone	May inhibit sexual interest and behavior in women (contained in many birth control pill and hormone replacement preparations) and in men (used to treat prostate cancer and hypersexual conditions)
Testosterone	Androgen (male hormone), which is the major sexual interest (libido) hormone in both women and men; secreted by the adrenal glands as well as the gonads throughout adult life; levels in men may be reduced by stress

27), and specific behavioral techniques, such as the squeeze technique and sensate focus exercises, are also useful.

   a. With the **squeeze technique** (used to treat premature ejaculation), the man is taught to identify the sensation that occurs just before the emission phase, when he can no longer prevent ejaculation. At this moment, the man asks his partner to exert pressure on the coronal ridge of the glans on both sides of the penis until the erection subsides.

   b. With **sensate focus exercises** (used to treat sexual desire, arousal, and orgasmic disorders), the patient is taught to increase his or her awareness of touch, sight, smell, and sound stimuli during sexual activity. In this way, psychological pressure to achieve orgasm is decreased.

3. The therapist may suggest **masturbation** (particularly for patients with orgasmic disorders) to help the patient experience sexual excitement and responsiveness and identify effective techniques for stimulation.

4. Some sexual dysfunctions in men are treated pharmacologically and surgically.

   a. Because they delay orgasm, **selective serotonin reuptake inhibitors** (SSRIs; e.g., fluoxetine) are used to **treat premature ejaculation.** Local anesthetics may also be applied cutaneously because they decrease sensation in the penis.

   b. **Sildenafil citrate (Viagra)** is an effective agent for treating male erectile disorder. It works by increasing the availability of cGMP, a vasodilator that helps maintain penile erection, when a man is sexually stimulated.

   c. Systemic administration of opioid antagonists (e.g., naltrexone) or systemic (e.g., yohimbine) or intracorporeal administration of **vasodilators** (e.g., papaverine, phentolamine) may be used to treat erectile dysfunction.

   d. Implantation of a prosthetic device is a surgical treatment for male erectile disorder.

   e. The treatment of comorbid drug and alcohol abuse should be undertaken.

II. SPECIAL SUBJECTS: ILLNESS, INJURY, AND AGING

A. Myocardial infarction (MI)

1. Men who have a history of MI often have erectile dysfunction. Both men and women who have a history of MI may have **decreased libido** because of medications and also fear that sexual activity will cause another heart attack.

2. Sexual activity can usually be resumed after MI when the patient can tolerate exercise that increases the **heart rate to 110–130 beats/minute** without severe shortness of breath or chest pain (i.e., exertion equal to climbing two flights of stairs).

3. **Sexual positions** that allow for the least exertion in the patient (i.e., the partner in the superior position) are the safest after MI.

B. Diabetes

1. **Erectile dysfunction is common** in men with diabetes; orgasm and ejaculation are less likely to be affected.

2. The major causes of erectile dysfunction in men with diabetes are **vascular changes** and **diabetic neuropathy** caused by damage to blood vessels and nerve tissue as a result of hyperglycemia.

3. Sildenafil citrate is often effective in diabetes-related erectile disorders.

C. Spinal cord injury

   1. Spinal cord injuries in men cause erectile and orgasmic dysfunction, retrograde ejaculation (into the bladder), reduced testosterone levels, and decreased fertility.

   2. Spinal cord injuries in women (much less common than in men) cause problems with vaginal lubrication, pelvic vasocongestion, and orgasm. Fertility is not usually affected.

D. Aging

   1. **Sexual interest usually does not change significantly with increasing age,** although opportunities for sexual expression may change due to a partner's illness or death.

   2. Age-related changes in men

   a. Need for more direct genital stimulation
   b. Increased time to achieve erection
   c. Decreased intensity of ejaculation
   d. Longer postejaculatory refractory period

   3. Age-related changes in women include vaginal thinning, shortening, and dryness. These changes can be **reversed with systemic or topical estrogen replacement therapy.**

III. DRUGS AND SEXUALITY

A. Prescription drugs that decrease sexuality

   1. Antihypertensives
   2. Antidepressants, particularly SSRIs **(serotonin may depress sexuality)**
   3. Antipsychotics, particularly D_2 receptor blockers

   a. **Dopamine may enhance sexuality;** its blockade may decrease sexual functioning.
   b. Prolactin levels increase as a result of dopamine blockade; this may in turn depress sexuality.

B. Drugs of abuse

   1. **Alcohol** and **marijuana** increase sexuality by **lowering inhibitions;** however, chronic alcohol use ultimately decreases both interest and performance.
   2. Amphetamines and cocaine increase sexuality by **stimulating dopaminergic systems.**
   3. Heroin and methadone decrease sexual interest and performance.

IV. PARAPHILIAS

A. Characteristics

   1. Preferential use of unusual objects of sexual desire or engagement in unusual sexual activity (Table 17-4) over a period of at least 6 months, causing impairment in occupational or social functioning.
   2. Unless they are recurrent and intense, paraphilic fantasies are not paraphilias, but rather are normal components of human sexuality.
   3. For the diagnosis of a paraphilia, a person must have fantasies, urges, and behaviors that preoccupy him and significantly interfere with his life.

B. Differential diagnosis, occurrence, and etiology

   1. The differential diagnosis includes dementia, schizophrenia, and situational difficulties (i.e., lack of appropriate partners).

Table 17-4.
Sexual Paraphilias

Paraphilia	Characteristics		Patient Snapshot
Exhibitionism	Revealing one's genitals to unsuspecting women so that they will be shocked		A 40-year-old man is arrested for exposing his penis to a woman on a bus.
Fetishism	Sexual preference for inanimate objects (e.g., women's shoes, rubber sheets)		A 34-year-old man always masturbates while stroking a rubber sheet.
Transvestic fetishism	Men gaining sexual gratification from wearing women's clothing, particularly underclothing		A 45-year-old man must wear women's lingerie to become aroused when he has intercourse with his wife.
Frotteurism	Obtaining sexual gratification by rubbing the penis against a woman who is nonconsenting and not aware		A 25-year-old man masturbates by rubbing against women in crowded buses.
Necrophilia	Obtaining sexual gratification through sexual activity with dead bodies		A 27-year-old man is convicted of murder for killing a woman to have sex with her corpse.
Pedophilia	Obtaining sexual gratification through fantasies or behaviors with children of the opposite or same sex; the most common paraphilia		A 39-year-old school principal is arrested when a 10-year-old girl complains that he told her to undress in his office so that he could take "nature" photographs of her.
Sexual sadism or masochism	Obtaining sexual pleasure from giving (sadism) or receiving (masochism) physical pain or humiliation		A 50-year-old bank president regularly pays a "dominatrix" to whip and embarrass him.
Telephone scatologia	Gaining sexual pleasure from making telephone calls to unsuspecting women and engaging them in conversations of a sexual nature		A 40-year-old man makes anonymous phone calls to teenage girls after school hours (but before their parents come home) so that he can talk to them about sex.
Voyeurism	Obtaining sexual pleasure from secretly watching people (often with binoculars) undressing or engaging in sexual activity		A 28-year-old man claiming to be a bird watcher is repeatedly arrested for looking into bedroom windows in his neighborhood.

2. Occurrence

    a. True paraphilias are uncommon. Pedophilia, voyeurism, and exhibitionism are the most frequently seen types.

    b. The occurrence of some paraphilias is unknown because they occur privately with consenting partners.

    c. Most paraphilias occur almost exclusively in men; however, pedophilia, sexual sadism, and sexual masochism are occasionally seen in women.

3. The etiology of paraphilias includes developmental psychological disturbances and possibly genetic and hormonal influences.

C. Treatment

    1. Psychological treatment includes psychotherapy that is psychoanalytically oriented and aversive conditioning (e.g., forming an association between mild electric shock and the preferred sexual activity; see Chapter 27).

    2. Pharmacologic treatment includes antiandrogens and female sex hormones, so-called **chemical castration,** for paraphilias that are characterized by hypersexuality. SSRIs are also useful.

D. Prognosis

    1. Predictors of a **good prognosis**

        a. Ability to have sexual intercourse without the paraphilia

        b. Guilt about the paraphilia

    2. Predictors of a **poor prognosis**

        a. Referral by law enforcement authorities rather than self-referral (most paraphilias are illegal, and arrests are common)

        b. Onset at a young age

V. GENDER IDENTITY DISORDER

A. Characteristics

    1. A 33-year-old woman says that she has always felt as if she was "a man in the body of a woman." She hates her breasts and feels as if her genitalia do not belong to her. She is sexually attracted to heterosexual women, is most comfortable wearing men's clothes, and wants to take male hormones and undergo a mastectomy and surgical sex reversal so that she can live as a man (i.e., have a male gender role).

    2. Commonly called "transsexuality," gender identity disorder is a person's subjective feeling that he has been born the wrong sex despite normal physiology; the person may take sex hormones or seek sex change surgery.

B. Differential diagnosis, occurrence, and etiology

    1. The differential diagnosis of gender identity disorder includes physiological hermaphroditism, schizophrenia, and persistent and marked distress about one's own sexual orientation (sexual disorder not otherwise specified).

    2. Although the overall prevalence is unknown, gender identity disorder is **more common in men.**

    3. Gender identity disorder **can often be diagnosed in childhood.**

    4. The etiology is not known, but it may be associated with abnormal prenatal levels of sex hormones.

C. Treatment and prognosis

    1. Many patients obtain sex hormones (often illegally) to acquire the secondary sex characteristics of the opposite sex (e.g., beard, breasts). Supportive psychotherapy is helpful.

    2. **Sex change surgery is rarely performed** now because in the past, depression and other psychological symptoms were not relieved after surgery.

    3. Gender identity disorder is often associated with lifelong distress, depression, and increased risk of suicide.

Table 17-5.

Biologic Sex, Gender Identity, Gender Role, and Sexual Orientation

Term	Definition
Biologic Sex	Genetic, hormonal, and anatomic factors that determine physiological sex
Gender identity	A person's sense of being male or female; develops by about 3 years of age
Gender role	The expression of one's gender identify in society (e.g., the type of clothing worn in public); may not agree with gender identity or biologic sex
Sexual Orientation	Choice of people of the same biologic sex (homosexual), the opposite biological sex (heterosexual), or both (bisexual) as sexual partners and love objects.

VI. HOMOSEXUALITY

A. Definition. Biologic sex, gender identity, gender role, and sexual orientation are defined in Table 17-5.

B. Characteristics

1. Homosexuality (i.e., having a gay or lesbian sexual orientation) (see Table 17-5) is **not considered a dysfunction** in the DSM-IV-TR.

   a. Homosexuality is a **normal variant** of sexual expression.

   b. **Distress about one's sexual preference** is considered a dysfunction. Formerly called "ego-dystonic homosexuality," it is currently diagnosed as a sexual disorder not otherwise specified.

2. Most gay or lesbian people have experienced heterosexual sex, and many have had children.

C. Occurrence and etiology

1. Homosexuality occurs in 3%–10% of men and 1%–5% of women but may be underreported. No significant ethnic differences are seen.

2. The etiology may be related to **alterations in prenatal hormone levels** (i.e., increased androgen levels in girls, decreased androgen levels in boys) that result in anatomic differences in certain hypothalamic nuclei. Sex hormone levels in adulthood are usually normal.

3. Genetic factors may also be involved.

D. Treatment and prognosis

1. Homosexual people who are distressed about their sexual orientation (or related social or economic problems) may become chronically depressed.

2. Psychological intervention can help the patient become comfortable with her sexual orientation; group therapy and specialized support groups may be helpful.

18

Obesity and Eating Disorders

I. OBESITY

A. Characteristics

    1. *(PATIENT SNAPSHOT)* A 20-year-old college student who is 5 feet, 9 inches tall and weighs 320 pounds says that he has been overweight all his life. He reports that his weight peaked at 380 pounds 2 years ago. He lost 100 pounds over the next year and regained 40 pounds during the last few months.

    2. Obesity is defined as being more than **20% over one's ideal weight** based on standard height and weight charts.

    3. Obesity is associated with increased risk of hypertension, cardiorespiratory problems, diabetes, and orthopedic problems.

    4. A subset of obese individuals has **binge eating disorder,** marked by discrete episodes of loss of control with greatly increased food intake.

B. Occurrence and etiology

    1. In the United States, at least **25% of adults are obese.**

    2. Obesity is more common in women and people in lower socioeconomic groups.

    3. Body weight tends to increase with age.

    4. **Genetic factors are important;** adult weight is closer to that of the biologic rather than the adoptive parents.

C. Treatment and prognosis

    1. Many commercial diet and weight loss programs are effective initially, but **most people regain the weight they have lost within 5 years.**

    2. Gastric stapling and other surgical techniques may be the only effective treatments for morbid obesity (> 100 pounds in excess of ideal body weight), even though they have significant morbidity and even mortality.

    3. Long-term weight loss is best achieved by a **combination of sensible dieting and exercise** tailored to the person's capabilities.

    4. **Overeaters Anonymous,** a 12-step self-help program based on Alcoholics Anonymous, can be helpful in maintaining weight loss.

    5. Pharmacologic treatments dexfenfluramine (Redux) and fenfluramine (Pondimin) have been taken off the market because their use led to heart valve abnormalities related to increased serotonin levels. The appetite suppressant **phentermine** (Ionamin), a sympathomimetic amine, is still used for some patients.

II. EATING DISORDERS: ANOREXIA NERVOSA AND BULIMIA NERVOSA

A. Overview

   1. Characteristics of patients with eating disorders

      a. Normal appetite

      b. Use of **compensatory mechanisms to avoid weight gain** (e.g., extreme dieting, vomiting, excessive exercising, abuse of laxatives)

      c. **Disturbance of body image** (e.g., unrealistic perception of looking fat)

      d. Menstrual cycle abnormalities

      e. Table 18-1 shows physical and psychological characteristics and patient snapshots for anorexia nervosa and bulimia nervosa.

   2. Occurrence and etiology

      a. Anorexia nervosa occurs in about 0.5% and bulimia nervosa in 1%–3% of women. Both disorders are ten times more common in women than in men.

      b. Eating disorders are more common in **late adolescence** and young adulthood; in anorexia nervosa, bimodal peak ages of onset are 14 and 18 years.

      c. Eating disorders are more common in **high academic achievers** and **higher socioeconomic groups.**

      d. Eating disorders are more prevalent in industrialized societies, where there is plenty of food.

      e. An important factor in these disorders is the **societal stereotype** that favors thin women.

      f. The onset is often associated with a **stressful life event,** like going away to college.

B. Anorexia nervosa

   1. Differential diagnosis

      a. General medical condition that causes weight loss

      b. Major depressive disorder that leads to poor appetite and weight loss

   2. Initial treatment

      a. Because starvation can lead to death, the goal of initial treatment is to **restore the patient's nutritional status.**

      b. If the patient's body weight is not too low, she can receive the initial treatment on an outpatient basis, with frequent office visits and regular weigh-ins. If the patient's body weight decreases to 20% or more below normal, she may be **admitted to the hospital** and treated until she achieves near-normal body weight.

   3. Pharmacologic and psychological treatment

      a. Amitriptyline (Elavil) and cyproheptadine (Periactin) are given to patients whose body weight is not dangerously low.

      b. Antipsychotics and selective serotonin reuptake inhibitors (SSRIs) may be effective in some patients.

      c. Because family dynamics, particularly mother–daughter relationships, are often a problem, the most effective form of psychotherapy is **family therapy.**

   4. Prognosis

      a. More than 10% of patients with anorexia nervosa **die** from starvation, electrolyte imbalance, or suicide.

      b. Some patients recover completely after a single episode. Others relapse frequently and have a chronic downhill course.

Table 18-1.
Anorexia Nervosa and Bulimia Nervosa: Patient Snapshots and Physical and Psychological Characteristics

Disorder	Patient Snapshot	Psychological Characteristics	Physical Characteristics
Anorexia nervosa	A 19-year-old gymnast says that she needs to lose 15 pounds to pursue a career in sports. She is 5 feet, 7 inches tall and weighs 95 pounds. Her mood is good. Findings on physical examination are normal except for excessive growth of downy body hair. She reports that she has not menstruated in more than 1 year.	Excessive dieting because of an overwhelming fear of being obese; refusal to eat despite normal appetite; abnormal behavior dealing with food (e.g., cutting food into very small pieces, simulating eating, cooking for others); conflicts about sexuality; lack of interest in sex; was a "perfect child" (e.g., obedient, good student); interfamily conflicts (e.g., patient's problem draws attention away from parental marital problem, an attempt to gain control to separate from the mother)	Weight loss (15% or more of normal body weight); amenorrhea (3 or more consecutive missed menstrual periods); metabolic acidosis; hypercholesterolemia; mild anemia and leukopenia; lanugo (downy body hair on the trunk); melanosis coli (blackened area of the colon because of laxative abuse)
Bulimia nervosa	A 22-year-old medical student has a parotid gland abscess. She is of normal weight for her height, but seems distressed when you question her about her eating habits.	Binge eating (in secret) of high-calorie foods usually followed by vomiting or other purging behavior to avoid weight gain (binge eating and purging also occurs in some patients with anorexia nervosa); poor self-image; serious concern about gaining weight; distress over the binge eating	Relatively normal body weight; esophageal varices caused by repeated vomiting; enamel erosion especially in anterior teeth due to dental caries caused by gastric acid in the mouth; swelling or infection of the parotid glands; scars and/or callouses on the dorsal surface of the hand from the teeth because the hand is used to induce gagging; electrolyte disturbances; menstrual irregularities

      c. Low body weight and obsession with food and eating often continue throughout life.

C. Bulimia nervosa

  1. Differential diagnosis

     a. Anorexia nervosa with binge eating and purging (body weight is far below normal)

     b. Kleine-Levin syndrome (episodic eating binges and hypersomnia without overconcern about body image or weight gain)

     c. Borderline personality disorder (poor impulse control, including impulsive eating)

  2. Treatment

     a. Psychological treatment includes cognitive and behavioral therapies.

     b. Pharmacologic treatment includes average to high doses of **antidepressants,** such as heterocyclics, selective serotonin reuptake inhibitors, and monoamine oxidase inhibitors. Combinations of cognitive therapy and antidepressants are most effective, even in the absence of depressive symptoms.

     c. Anticonvulsants and lithium are used to treat patients who have comorbid bipolar mood disorders.

  3. The course can be intermittent or chronic; many patients show diminished symptoms at long-term follow up.

19

Impulse-Control Disorders

I. OVERVIEW

A. Patients with impulse-control disorders are **unable to resist** engaging in behavior that is harmful to themselves or other people.

B. Patients usually experience **increased tension** before the behavior and **relief** or pleasure after the behavior is completed.

C. Table 19-1 shows the occurrence, etiology, treatment, and prognosis of the impulse-control disorders: kleptomania, pyromania, intermittent explosive disorder, pathological gambling, and trichotillomania.

II. KLEPTOMANIA

A. A 30-year-old professional tennis player is caught taking an inexpensive radio from a store without paying for it. He has been caught shoplifting twice before.

B. Kleptomania is the **impulse to take things without paying for them** (even if they are affordable). Taking, rather than owning, the object is the intent.

C. The theft is not an act of defiance or of anger.

D. **Differential diagnosis**

    1. Stealing during a manic episode

    2. Stealing for actual gain

    3. Faking kleptomania (malingering) to avoid prosecution for stealing

    4. Conduct disorder in children (younger than 18 years of age) and antisocial personality disorder in adults (18 years of age and older), both of which are associated with many other behavioral problems

III. INTERMITTENT EXPLOSIVE DISORDER

A. A 34-year-old man is arrested for leaving his car and physically attacking another motorist stopped at a traffic light. A witness reports that the had victim cut the man off at the previous light.

B. Intermittent explosive disorder is characterized by episodes in which the patient **loses self-control** and attacks another person without adequate cause. It was formerly called "episodic dyscontrol syndrome."

Table 19-1.
Impulse-Control Disorders

Disorder	Occurrence	Etiology	Treatment	Prognosis
Kleptomania	Present in less than 5% of shoplifters; more common in patients with bulimia nervosa	Family dysfunction in childhood; precipitated by life stress	Aversive conditioning (see Chapter 27); selective serotonin reuptake inhibitors (SSRIs)	Chronic; arrest, legal punishment, and shame are common
Pyromania	More common in men; often seen in conduct disorder in childhood (see Chapter 4)	Family problems in childhood	SSRIs	Good prognosis for children; poor prognosis for adults
Intermittent explosive disorder	More common in men; familial pattern; onset usually in the late teens or twenties	Decreased serotonergic activity reflected in reduced levels of 5-hydroxyindoleacetic acid (5-HIAA), resulting in impulsivity	Anticonvulsants (e.g., carbamazepine), SSRIs	Progresses in severity until middle age; relationship and occupational problems are common
Pathological gambling	Seen in up to 3% of adults; higher in late teens and early 20s; onset at a later age in women than in men	Associated with loss of parent before or during adolescence, childhood attention-deficit/ hyperactivity disorder, and major depressive disorder	Gamblers Anonymous (12-step program modeled after Alcoholics Anonymous) is most effective	Chronic and lifelong; financial problems may occur and lead to theft or bankruptcy
Trichotillomania	More common in women; begins in childhood	Life stress, depression	SSRIs, antipsychotics [e.g., pimozide (Orap)]	Chronic; may last for years

C. Patients often have soft neurologic findings and nonspecific evidence of cerebral dysfunction.

D. Differential diagnosis

  1. Alcohol or drug intoxication

  2. Loss of touch with reality (e.g., psychosis or dementia)

  3. Conduct disorder

  4. Antisocial personality disorder

  5. Dissociative disorder (e.g., dissociative symptoms occur in "amok," a single episode of explosive behavior seen most commonly in Southeast Asia)

IV. PYROMANIA

A. A 29-year-old volunteer fireman is arrested after he is found setting fires in the hallway of his apartment building.

B. Pyromania is characterized by **repetitive fire setting** and overwhelming interest in and attraction to fires.

C. Individuals with this disorder sometimes seek situations in which they can be involved with fires (e.g., they become volunteer firefighters).

D. Differential diagnosis

  1. Normal curiosity about fire

  2. Arson (i.e., insurance gain for losses due to fire)

  3. Impaired judgment because of another mental condition (e.g., mental retardation)

V. PATHOLOGICAL GAMBLING

A. A 60-year-old woman is afraid to tell her husband that her credit cards are at their maximum because she lost more than $10,000 gambling in a casino. She ran up debt in this way twice before.

B. Patients have an **overwhelming need to gamble** that negatively affects family and work relationships.

C. The differential diagnosis includes a manic episode in which there is obvious elevation of mood.

VI. TRICHOTILLOMANIA

A. A 29-year-old woman wears a wig because she has pulled out all of the hair on the back of her head.

B. Patients with trichotillomania have a **need to pull out their hair.** The result is obvious hair loss. Some also show tricophagia (hair eating), resulting in bezoars (hair balls), which can obstruct the bowel.

C. Differential diagnosis

  1. Alopecia (hair loss) caused by a medical condition

  2. Obsessive-compulsive disorder, which is not limited to one compulsion

20
Adjustment Disorders

I. CHARACTERISTICS AND DIFFERENTIAL DIAGNOSIS

A. People who experience a stressful life event show either a normal response (e.g., normal grief reaction) or a **maladaptive response** (e.g., adjustment disorder, acute stress disorder, brief psychotic disorder; Table 20-1).

B. Differential diagnosis

1. The conditions included in the differential diagnosis of adjustment disorder are distinguished in part by the **nature of the stressful life event.**

a. In adjustment disorder or in a normal grief reaction, the stressor is experienced by many people at some point (e.g., financial problems, serious illness). The stressor may also be quite severe.

b. In the anxiety disorders—acute stress disorder and posttraumatic stress disorder (PTSD)—the stressor is intense, often life-threatening, and unlikely to be experienced by most people (e.g., combat, rape, assault).

c. In brief psychotic disorder, the stressor may be mild or severe, but the response involves a loss of touch with reality.

2. These conditions are distinguished also by the patient's **social, academic, or occupational functioning during and after the stressor.**

a. The patient who has a normal response to life stress or a normal grief reaction functions relatively normally.

b. The patient with adjustment disorder, acute stress disorder, PTSD, or brief psychotic disorder cannot function normally.

II. SUBTYPES OF ADJUSTMENT DISORDER

A. With depressed mood. Patients have symptoms of depression (e.g., hopelessness, sadness, tearfulness).

B. With anxiety. Patients have symptoms of anxiety (e.g., tremor, gastrointestinal symptoms).

C. With mixed anxiety and depressed mood. Patients have symptoms of both depression and anxiety.

D. With disturbance of conduct. Patients violate social norms (e.g., fighting, stealing).

E. With mixed disturbance of emotions and conduct. Patients have conduct disturbances in addition to depression or anxiety.

F. Unspecified. Patients have maladaptive responses to psychosocial stress (e.g., inhibited social interactions, problems at work).

Table 20-1.
Differential Diagnosis of Adjustment Disorder

Disorder	Characteristics		Patient Snapshot
Adjustment disorder	Emotional symptoms that start within 3 months and end within 6 months of exposure to a psychosocial stressor (e.g., divorce, financial difficulties, retirement); impairment in occupational, academic, or social functioning	PATIENT SNAPSHOT	Four months after his parents' divorce, a 10-year-old boy seems sad at home most of the time, loses interest in playing with his friends, and begins to do poorly in school.
Normal grief reaction (bereavement; see Chapter 6)	Expected strong emotional response, usually sadness, after a loss (e.g., death of a loved one, abortion, stillbirth, loss of a body part)	PATIENT SNAPSHOT	Six months after a mastectomy, a 48-year-old woman feels sad for a few minutes each evening and often wakes before her alarm goes off; however, she continues to do well in her job and enjoys social interactions with coworkers and family.
Acute stress disorder (see Chapter 14)	Multiple psychological symptoms (e.g., anxiety, withdrawal, dissociation) lasting 2 days to 4 weeks within a month after exposure to an intense psychosocial stressor; impairment in functioning; may become chronic and last for years	PATIENT SNAPSHOT	Three weeks after a mugging in which her shoulder was fractured, a 65-year-old woman cannot sleep, shows little interest in her usual activities, and shows an intense startle response whenever she hears a loud noise.
Posttraumatic stress disorder (see Chapter 14)	Multiple psychological symptoms lasting more than 4 weeks after exposure to an intense psychosocial stressor; impairment in functioning; may become chronic and last for years	PATIENT SNAPSHOT	Three years after a mugging in which her shoulder was fractured, a 68-year-old woman remains hypervigilant and anxious. She has frequent nightmares about the event that interrupt her sleep and leave her chronically tired.
Brief psychotic disorder (see Chapter 12)	One or more psychotic symptoms occurring over a period of more than 1 day but less than 1 month, followed by a full return to the premorbid level of functioning	PATIENT SNAPSHOT	During exam week, a 20-year-old college student begins to suspect that her roommate is trying to poison her (a delusion). She returns to normal after exams.

III. OCCURRENCE AND ETIOLOGY

A. Occurrence

   1. Adjustment disorder is **common** and is diagnosed in 2%–8% of children, adolescents, and the elderly; it is present in 10%–30% of mental health outpatients.

   2. It is more common in disadvantaged populations, possibly because of economic stress.

   3. There is no gender difference in adjustment disorder in children. In adults, women are more likely to be diagnosed than men.

B. Etiology

   1. The etiology of adjustment disorder is **life stress,** although the intensity of the symptoms does not always correlate with the severity of the stressor.

   2. Adjustment disorder in adulthood is correlated with **poor tolerance of frustration** and stress because of the loss of a parent or a poor relationship with the parents during early life.

IV. TREATMENT

A. The most effective treatment is **supportive psychotherapy** to help the patient adapt to the stressful event and to provide alternative coping strategies.

B. Other treatments include **group therapy** (e.g., with other laid-off workers).

C. Pharmacotherapy is used to treat associated insomnia, depression, or anxiety.

V. PROGNOSIS

A. If the stressor is acute, adjustment disorder has a short latency to onset and a brief duration (e.g., no more than six months).

B. If the stressor is chronic (e.g., a chronic medical illness), adjustment disorder may continue for a longer period (e.g., six months after the termination of the stressor).

21

Personality Disorders

I. DEFINITION AND CATEGORIES

A. Definition. Personality disorders (PDs) are pervasive, fixed, **inappropriate patterns of relating to others** that cause **social and occupational impairment.**

B. Categories

    1. The categories of PDs are paranoid, schizoid, schizotypal, histrionic, narcissistic, antisocial, borderline, avoidant, obsessive-compulsive, dependent, and passive-aggressive.

    2. **The DSM-IV-TR** classifies PDs as **Cluster A, Cluster B,** or **Cluster C** based on shared characteristics and familial genetic associations. Table 21-1 shows patient snapshots and characteristics of each PD.

    3. People with atypical personality traits or combinations of abnormal personality traits are diagnosed as having personality disorder not otherwise specified (NOS).

II. GENERAL CHARACTERISTICS, DIFFERENTIAL DIAGNOSIS, OCCURRENCE, ETIOLOGY, TREATMENT, AND PROGNOSIS

A. General characteristics

    1. Patients with PDs typically **have limited insight** (i.e., they are not aware that they are the cause of their own problems).

    2. They **do not seek psychological help** unless compelled by others.

    3. They **do not have a frank psychosis.**

    4. They usually **do not have disabling psychiatric symptoms** (e.g., anxiety, depression), except when the PD leads to conflict with others.

    5. Age of onset

        a. For a diagnosis to be made, the PD **must be present by early adulthood.**

        b. Antisocial PD cannot be diagnosed until the patient is at least 18 years old; before age 18, the diagnosis is conduct disorder (see Chapter 4).

B. Differential diagnosis. Table 21-2 shows the differential diagnosis for PDs.

C. Occurrence and etiology

    1. Each individual PD affects approximately 1% of the population, although many patients have features of more than one PD. Histrionic, dependent, and schizotypal PDs are more common; schizoid PD is less common.

Table 21-1.

Characteristics and Patient Snapshots of the DSM-IV-TR Personality Disorders

Personality Disorder	Characteristics		Patient Snapshot
CLUSTER A: Peculiar; fears social relationships; genetic or familial association with psychotic illnesses			
Paranoid	Distrustful, suspicious, litigious; attributes responsibility for own problems to others		A 45-year-old hospital aide says that she was laid off because she worked too hard and made her supervisor look lazy. She says that when the same thing happened in a previous job, she filed a lawsuit against that hospital.
Schizoid	Long-standing pattern of voluntary social withdrawal without psychosis		The parents of a 26-year-old man say that they are concerned about him because he has no friends and spends most of his time hiking in the woods. You examine him and find that he is content with his solitary life and has no evidence of a formal thought disorder.
Schizotypal	Peculiar appearance, magical thinking, odd thought patterns and behavior without psychosis; not uncommonly patients also have major depressive disorder		An oddly dressed 32-year-old woman says that she likes to walk in the woods because the birds communicate with her. She says that she never goes out on Thursdays, however, because they are "dangerous days." She has few friends.
CLUSTER B: Emotional, inconsistent, or dramatic; genetic or familial association with mood disorders, substance abuse, and somatoform disorders			
Histrionic	Theatrical, extroverted, emotional, sexually provocative, "life of the party"; cannot maintain intimate relationships; in men, "Don Juan" dress and behavior		A 28-year-old man comes to your office dressed in a black velvet beret and a cape lined with red satin. He reports that his mild sore throat felt like "a hot poker" when he swallowed and says that he feels so warm that he "must have a fever of at least 106°."
Narcissistic	Pompous, with a sense of special entitlement; lacks empathy for others		A 38-year-old man asks you to refer him to a physician who attended a top medical school. He says that he knows you will not be offended because you understand that he is "better" than your other patients.

(continued)

Table 21-1.—*Continued*
Characteristics and Patient Snapshots of the DSM-IV-TR Personality Disorders

Personality Disorder	Characteristics		Patient Snapshot
Antisocial	Refuses to conform to social norms, shows no concern for others, and does not learn from experience; associated with conduct disorder in childhood and criminal behavior in adulthood ("psychopaths" or "sociopaths")		A 35-year-old man brags that he has been sexually assaulting women ever since high school, but has never been caught. He has often been unemployed and has been arrested for shoplifting several times.
Borderline	Erratic, unstable behavior and mood; boredom; feelings of aloneness (i.e., feeling alone in the world, not merely loneliness); impulsiveness, suicide attempts, and mini-psychotic episodes (i.e., brief periods of loss of contact with reality); self-mutilation (cutting or burning oneself); often comorbid with mood disorders and eating disorders		A 20-year-old female college student tells you that because she was afraid to be alone again, she tried to commit suicide after a man with whom she had had two dates did not call her again. After your interview, she tells you that all of the other doctors she has seen were terrible and that you are the only doctor who has ever understood her problems (use of "splitting" as a defense mechanism; see Table 21-3).
CLUSTER C: Fearful, anxious; genetic or familial association with anxiety disorders			
Avoidant	Timid, sensitive to rejection, and socially withdrawn; feelings of inferiority		A 35-year-old woman who works as a laboratory assistant lives with her elderly mother and rarely socializes. She reports that when coworkers ask her to join them for lunch, she refuses because she is afraid that they will not like her.
Obsessive-compulsive	Perfectionistic, orderly, stubborn, indecisive, feelings of imperfection		A 33-year-old man reports that each night he creates a detailed schedule of his activities for the next day. He tells you that his wife of 6 months recently moved out because she could not conform to his rigid rules.
Dependent	Allows other people to make decisions and assume responsibility for them because of poor self-confidence; may be abused by domestic partner		A 32-year-old woman says that her husband is angry because she calls him at the office many times each day to ask him to make trivial, everyday decisions for her.

(*continued*)

Table 21-1.—*Continued*
Characteristics and Patient Snapshots of the DSM-IV-TR Personality Disorders

Personality Disorder	Characteristics		Patient Snapshot
Passive-aggressive	Procrastinates; inefficient; outward compliance, but inward defiance (no longer an official DSM-IV-TR diagnosis)	PATIENT SNAPSHOT	Two weeks after a 50-year-old overweight, hypertensive woman agreed to start an exercise program, she gained 4 pounds. She reports that she has not exercised yet because "the gym was so crowded that I couldn't get in."

2. PDs have a genetic association with some psychiatric disorders. These disorders are more common in relatives of patients with PDs than in the general population (see Table 21-1).

3. Psychological factors may also be implicated (e.g., overuse of maladaptive or inappropriate defense mechanisms; Table 21-3).

D. Treatment and prognosis

1. Pharmacologic treatment is of limited use in PDs, except for borderline PD, where antipsychotics or antidepressants may be necessary.

   a. Medication is used to treat associated target symptoms (e.g., depression, anxiety, mini-psychotic episodes).

   b. Medication must be prescribed cautiously (especially benzodiazepines) because many patients with PDs have a **high potential for addiction.**

2. Individual and group psychotherapy and self-help groups may be useful.

3. PDs are chronic and lifelong.

Table 21-2.
Differential Diagnoses of the Personality Disorders

Personality Disorder	Differential Diagnosis	How the condition in the differential diagnosis varies from the personality disorder
Paranoid	• Delusional disorder (see Chapter 12), paranoid type schizophrenia (see Chapter 11), mood disorder with psychotic features (see Chapter 13)	Frank or enduring psychotic symptoms (e.g., delusions)
Schizoid	• Delusional disorder, schizophrenia	Frank or enduring psychotic symptoms
	• Asperger disorder, autistic disorder (see Chapter 5)	Stereotyped behavior patterns, impaired social communication
Schizotypal	• Delusional disorder, schizophrenia, mood disorder with psychotic features	Frank or enduring psychotic symptoms

(continued)

Table 21-2.—*Continued*
Differential Diagnoses of the Personality Disorders

Personality Disorder	Differential Diagnosis	How the condition in the differential diagnosis varies from the personality disorder
Histrionic	• Borderline personality disorder	Chronic feelings of boredom and emptiness; suicidal behavior
	• Narcissistic personality disorder	Feelings of superiority
	• Dependent personality disorder	Not characterized by flamboyance or an overly emotional state
	• Hypomanic episode in bipolar II or cyclothymic disorder (see Chapter 13)	Symptoms dissipate when the episode ends
Narcissistic	• Histrionic, personality disorder, borderline personality disorder	Instability and emotionality
	• Obsessive-compulsive personality disorder	Feelings of imperfection
Antisocial	• Criminal behavior	Includes obvious gain
	• Substance abuse (see Chapter 10)	May involve stealing to obtain money for drugs
	• Narcissistic personality disorder	Needs admiration from others
	• Paranoid personality disorder	May be characterized by illegal behavior to obtain revenge
	• Hypomanic episode in bipolar II or cyclothymic disorder	Symptoms dissipate when the episode ends
Borderline	• Histrionic, paranoid, and narcissistic personality disorders	Do not include self-destructive behavior or feelings of aloneness
Avoidant	• Social phobia (see Chapter 14)	Significant symptoms of anxiety in social situations
	• Dependent personality disorder	Primarily seeks care from others
	• Schizoid personality disorder	Content with little social contact
	• Atypical depression	Does not include sensitivity to rejection
Obsessive-compulsive	• Obsessive-compulsive anxiety disorder (OCD)	Presence of actual obsessions and compulsions; anxiety occurs if they are not carried out (see Chapter 14)
Dependent	• Depression	More episodic, less chronic
Passive-aggressive	• Oppositional defiant disorder	More directly defiant; usually seen in children
	• Subordinate who must reluctantly accept an assignment by a superior	Behavior results from the need to retain employment

Table 21-3.

Defense Mechanisms and Other Psychodynamic Mechanisms Used by Patients With DSM-IV-TR Personality Disorders

Personality Disorder	Psychodynamic Mechanisms (see Chapter 26)
Paranoid	• Denial: psychologically blocking out intolerable facts about reality • Projection: attributing one's unconscious, unacceptable impulses to others
Histrionic	• Repression: pushing unacceptable feelings into the unconscious • Regression: adopting childlike behavioral patterns • Somatization (see Chapter 15)
Narcissistic	• Denial • Displacement: transferring emotions from an unacceptable to a tolerable person or situation • Poor ego functioning
Antisocial	• Inadequate superego functioning
Borderline	• Denial • Displacement • Splitting: seeing others as either all bad or all good • Poor ego functioning
Avoidant	• Displacement • Avoidance • Regression
Obsessive-compulsive	• Isolation of affect: neither experiencing nor expressing emotions associated with stressful events • Rationalization: giving seemingly reasonable explanations for unacceptable feelings • Intellectualization: explaining away unwanted emotions • Undoing: attempting to reverse past actions by current actions
Dependent	• Regression • Avoidance
Passive-aggressive	• Reaction formation: denying unacceptable feelings and adopting opposite attitudes and behavior

22
Psychosomatic Medicine

I. PSYCHOLOGICAL FACTORS THAT AFFECT MEDICAL CONDITIONS

A. Vulnerable systems of the body. The cardiovascular, gastrointestinal, respiratory, genitourinary, musculoskeletal, endocrine, dermatologic, immunologic, and neurologic systems are affected by psychological factors.

B. Psychological factors that may initiate or exacerbate symptoms of medical illness

    1. Chronic or severe **life stress** (e.g., poverty, relationship problems)

    2. Poor health behavior (e.g., overeating, lack of exercise, smoking)

    3. Emotional symptoms (e.g., depression, anxiety)

    4. Maladaptive personality styles (e.g., dependency, type A behavior; Table 22-1)

C. Physiologic effects of stress

    1. Activation of the **autonomic nervous system,** which leads to cardiovascular and respiratory changes

    2. Altered levels of neurotransmitters (e.g., serotonin, norepinephrine), which lead to changes in mood and behavior

    3. Increased release of adrenocorticotropic hormone (ACTH), which leads to the release of cortisol, ultimately resulting in **depression of the immune system** as measured by:

        a. Decreased lymphocyte response to mitogens
        b. Impaired function of natural killer (NK) cells

D. Stressful life events

    1. The amount of stress in a patient's life may be directly related to the likelihood of medical and psychiatric illness.

    2. The **Social Readjustment Rating Scale** by Holmes and Rahe (which also includes "happy" events) ranks the effects of life events (Table 22-2). Events with high scores require the most "social readjustment."

    3. Social readjustment increases the risk of medical and psychiatric illness; in studies by Holmes and Rahe, 80% of patients with a score of 300 points in a given year became ill during the next year.

    4. Although the death of a spouse had the highest score (100 points), other life stressors not considered by Holmes and Rahe (e.g., death of a child, suicide of a spouse) may be even more stressful.

Table 22-1.
Personality Characteristics Associated With Medical Conditions

Medical Condition	Associated Personality Characteristic		Patient Snapshot
Coronary artery disease, hypertension	Type A personality, which is characterized primarily by time pressure (i.e., feeling rushed most of the time), and competitiveness, and may also include hostility; hostility in particular may be associated with coronary artery disease		A 38-year-old salesman who is hospitalized for a myocardial infarction says that he never takes time for lunch or a day off because he wants to be named "salesman of the year." He becomes angry when you tell him that he may need to slow down, and he signs out of the hospital against medical advice.
Bronchial asthma	Excessive dependency		A 14-year-old boy with bronchial asthma refuses to leave the house for any reason unless a parent accompanies him.
Cancer	Inability to express feelings, bereavement		A 65-year-old man who was recently diagnosed with renal carcinoma tells you that he has never recovered from the death of his youngest daughter.
Migraine headache, ulcerative colitis	Obsessive-compulsive personality type		As you are about to examine him, a 40-year-old lawyer with ulcerative colitis says that he must call his office.
Obesity	Regression (i.e., return to developmentally earlier patterns of behavior)		A 28-year-old overweight woman says that whenever she becomes upset or tense, she eats cookies and drinks hot chocolate, which were her favorite treats in childhood.

II. PERSONALITY CHARACTERISTICS LINKED TO MEDICAL CONDITIONS.
Certain medical conditions are associated with specific personality characteristics (Table 22-1).

III. MEDICAL CONDITIONS THAT CAUSE PSYCHIATRIC SYMPTOMS. Some
medical conditions have predictable psychiatric manifestations such as anxiety, depression, or personality changes (Table 22-3).

Table 22-2.
Magnitude of Stress Associated With Selected Life Events According to the Holmes and Rahe Social Readjustment Rating Scale

Life Event	Stress Points	Patient Snapshot
Death of a spouse	100	A 65-year-old man is admitted to the hospital after a stroke. During the last year, both his wife (100 points) and his older brother (63 points) died. After his wife's death, he retired from his job (45 points) and moved to a luxury apartment (20 points), which required taking out a new mortgage (31 points). During the move, he fell and fractured his hip and was hospitalized for 6 weeks (53 points).
Divorce	73	
Death of a close family member	63	
Serious illness or injury	53	
Marriage	50	
Retirement or loss of job	45	
Birth of a child	39	
Assuming a large loan or mortgage	31	Total = 312 points
Changing residence	20	

Table 22-3.
Psychiatric Symptoms Associated With Medical Conditions

Psychiatric Symptom	Associated Medical Conditions		Patient Snapshot
Anxiety	Anemias, cardiac arrhythmias and mitral valve prolapse, chronic infections with fever, hyperaldrenalism (Cushing disease), hyperthyroidism, hypoglycemia or hyperglycemia, pheochromocytoma, pulmonary disease		A 28-year-old woman with no history of psychiatric disorder experiences palpitations and acute anxiety. Physical examination shows bulging eyes (exophthalmus) and a neck mass (enlarged thyroid gland). A blood test reveals hyperthyroidism.
Depression	AIDS; brain lesion, particularly in the left frontal lobe; collagen-vascular disease [(e.g., systemic lupus erythematosus (SLE)]; chronic pain (e.g., headache); hypoadrenalism (Addison disease) and Cushing disease; hypothyroidism; hypoparathyroidism and hyperparathyroidism; Huntington disease; infectious illness (e.g., influenza, mononucleosis); multiple sclerosis; pancreatic and other gastrointestinal cancers; Parkinson disease; vitamin deficiency		A 67-year-old physician with no history of psychiatric disorder suddenly becomes severely depressed. Three months later he is diagnosed with pancreatic cancer.
Personality changes	Brain infection, neoplasm, or trauma; dementia; delirium; Huntington disease; temporal lobe epilepsy; tertiary syphilis; Wilson disease (explosive anger)		A 75-year-old woman with no history of psychiatric illness becomes unusually irritable and suspicious of her husband. Four months later she is diagnosed with Alzheimer dementia.
Mania, psychotic symptoms	AIDS, acute intermittent porphyria, Cushing disease, Huntington disease, multiple sclerosis, neoplasm, SLE		After a 1-week trip to the Caribbean, a 35-year-old woman begins to believe that the television newscasters are publicly discussing her behavior. Three weeks later, she is diagnosed with SLE. (Note: Sun exposure exacerbates the symptoms of SLE.)

23

Medication-Induced Psychiatric Symptoms

I. PSYCHOTROPIC AGENTS. Antidepressants, antipsychotics, antianxiety agents, and stimulants cause psychiatric symptoms in some patients (Table 23-1).

Table 23-1.
Psychiatric Symptoms Caused by Psychotropic Agents

Class of Agent	Psychiatric Symptoms		Patient Snapshot
Antipsychotics	Agitation, confusion, delirium, insomnia, sedation, sexual dysfunction		A 25-year-old man who has schizophrenia and recently started taking haloperidol is now distractible and confused.
Antidepressants	Agitation, confusion, delirium, insomnia, sedation, sexual dysfunction, precipitation of a manic episode in a patient who may have bipolar disorder		Two weeks after she begins taking antidepressant medication, a 32-year-old woman appears hyperexcited, shows flight of ideas (rapid sequence of thoughts) and says that she communicates directly with God each morning (precipitation of a manic episode).
Antianxiety agents	Sedation, decreased concentration		A 65-year-old woman who takes temazepam (30 mg/day) for sleep says that she has difficulty waking up in the morning and cannot concentrate on even simple tasks.
Stimulants (e.g., methylphenidate, dextroamphetamine)	Anxiety, insomnia, paranoid psychotic symptoms		A mother reports that her 9-year-old son, who has attention-deficit hyperactivity disorder and is taking methylphenidate, gets out of bed repeatedly during the night and seems agitated during the day.

II. NONPSYCHOTROPIC AGENTS. Some drugs that are used to treat medical conditions can precipitate psychiatric symptoms (Table 23-2).

Table 23-2.

Psychiatric Symptoms Caused by Nonpsychotropic Agents

Class of Agent	Specific Medications	Psychiatric Symptoms
Analgesics	Pentazocine, propoxyphene	Psychotic symptoms
Antiarrhythmics	Procainamide, quinidine	Confusion, occasionally delirium
Antiasthmatics	Albuterol, terbutaline, theophylline	Confusion, anxiety
Antibiotics	Antitubercular agents (e.g., isoniazid) Chloramphenicol, metronidazole Tetracycline Nitrofurantoin	Psychotic symptoms (e.g., paranoia), memory loss Confusion, depression, irritability Depression Confusion, headache, sleepiness
Anticholinergics	Atropine, scopolamine, trihexyphenidyl, benztropine	Drowsiness, agitation; poor concentration in low doses; psychotic symptoms in high doses (atropine toxic psychosis)
Anticonvulsants	Phenacemide, phenytoin	Mood symptoms, confusion, psychotic symptoms (less common)
Antihistamines	Diphenhydramine, hydroxyzine Phenylephrine, phenylpropanolamine	Sleepiness Psychotic symptoms, anxiety
Antihypertensives	Guanethidine, clonidine, methyldopa, some diuretics β-blockers (e.g., propranolol) Reserpine	Mild depression, fatigue, sexual dysfunction Depression, fatigue, psychotic symptoms (less common) Severe depression, confusion
Antineoplastics	Fluorouracil	Confusion, disorientation, mood changes
Antiparkinson agents	L-dopa	Anxiety, psychosis, delirium, mania, depression
Cardiac glycosides	Digitalis	Mild depression, fatigue; delirium is associated with toxicity (particularly in the elderly)
Calcium channel blockers	Nifedipine, verapamil	Depression
Hypoglycemics	Insulin	Anxiety, confusion

(*continued*)

Table 23-2.—*Continued*

Psychiatric Symptoms Caused by Nonpsychotropic Agents

Class of Agent	Specific Medications	Psychiatric Symptoms
Nonsteroidal anti-inflammatory agents	Salicylates	Euphoria, depression, confusion (in very high doses)
	Indomethacin	Confusion, dizziness, psychotic symptoms, depression (less common)
	Phenylbutazone	Anxiety
Peptic ulcer drugs	Cimetidine	Depression, psychotic symptoms
Steroid hormones	Androgens	Aggressiveness, agitation
	Corticosteroids (use)	Hypomania, euphoria,
	Corticosteroids (abrupt withdrawal)	Depression, confusion, psychotic symptoms; fatigue, symptoms such as headache and vomiting imitating a brain tumor ("pseudotumor cerebri")
	Progestins	Depression, fatigue
	Thyroid hormones [e.g., triiodothyronine (T_3), thyroxine (T_4)]	Anxiety, psychotic symptoms

24

Consultation–Liaison Psychiatry

I. OVERVIEW

A. Consultation–liaison (CL) **psychiatrists treat psychiatric problems in medical patients.**

B. Table 24-1 describes the major problems treated by CL psychiatrists. Other commonly treated complaints include anxiety, sleep disorders, and disorientation, often as a result of delirium (see Chapter 9).

C. In addition to recommending specific psychotropic medications, CL psychiatrists provide the following psychosocial interventions:

1. Identify and organize the patient's **social support systems.**

2. Address the immediate problem through short-term, **dynamic psychotherapy** (see Chapter 26).

3. Develop a plan to deal with the patient's social or occupational problems.

II. PATIENTS AT RISK.
Hospitalized patients who are at the greatest risk for psychological problems include patients with acquired immune deficiency syndrome (AIDS), patients on renal dialysis, patients who are undergoing surgery, and patients who are being treated in the intensive care unit (ICU) or coronary care unit (CCU).

A. Patients with AIDS

1. Reasons for psychological risk in patients with AIDS

    a. The illness is **potentially fatal.**

    b. Patients may experience **guilt** because they engaged in behavior that led to the illness (e.g., sex with multiple partners, intravenous drug abuse) and may have given the virus to others.

    c. They must deal with others' **fears of contagion.**

    d. Homosexual patients may be forced to **"come out"** (reveal their sexual orientation) to others.

2. Psychological counseling can reduce psychological and medical risk.

B. Patients undergoing renal dialysis

1. Patients on renal dialysis are at increased risk for psychological problems, in part because they must depend on other people and on machines.

2. The most common psychological problems in these patients are **depression, suicide,** and **sexual dysfunction.**

3. Psychological and medical risk can be reduced through the use of in-home dialysis units, which cause less disruption of the patient's life.

Table 24-1.
Common Psychological Problems in Hospitalized Medical Patients

Problem	Patient Snapshot	Intervention
Noncompliance with medical advice or treatment	A patient whose father and grandfather died of prostate cancer says that he cannot take a prostate-specific antigen test because "the needle will leave a mark."	• Identify the real reason why the patient refuses to undergo the test (probably fear of a positive result). Address the patient's fear of the illness
Refusal to consent to needed medical or surgical procedures	Even though the fetus will die if she does not consent, a woman in labor who seems to be competent refuses to allow a cesarean delivery. Note: Competent pregnant women, like all competent adults, can refuse medical treatment, even if the fetus will be harmed or die as a result.	• Identify the reason for the patient's refusal to consent and address it. • Assess the patient's ability to give or to withhold informed consent, that is, whether she understands the risks and benefits of the cesarean delivery and what will happen if she refuses to consent. • If she is competent to give informed consent and she still refuses, deliver the child vaginally. • If there is any question about the patient's capacity to consent, only a judge can make a final legal determination of competency (see Chapter 29).
Depression, suicidal threats	A patient with AIDS says that as soon as he is released from the hospital, he will kill himself.	• Assess the seriousness of the threat. • If it is serious, suggest that the patient remain in the hospital voluntarily. • Transfer the patient to the psychiatric service if necessary. • If he does not consent, hold the patient involuntarily (see Chapter 29).
Resistance to treatment for medical complications of substance abuse	A middle-aged man who is being treated on the medical floor for advanced liver cirrhosis has been observed sneaking wine onto the floor.	• Provide non-judgmental substance abuse counseling. Arrange for the patient to attend an AA group in the hospital.

(continued)

Table 24-1.—*Continued*

Common Psychological Problems in Hospitalized Medical Patients

Problem	Patient Snapshot	Intervention
Chronic psychiatric illness in a patient admitted for other reasons	A chronic schizophrenic patient, who is hospitalized for uterine bleeding during the first trimester of her pregnancy, insists that the blood is a sign from God that the baby will be the next Messiah.	• Assist the treating obstetrician in her management of the patient, recommending psychotropic agents with the least teratogenic risk.
Medical complications of psychotropic agents	A patient who was transferred to the medical floor after developing neuroleptic malignant syndrome (NMS) (see Chapter 11), secondary to haloperidol, is medically improved but still psychotic	• Work with the internist to develop a new management plan, with the aim of treating the psychotic symptoms, but minimizing the risk of recurrence of NMS.
Medical complications of a suicide attempt	A patient who was transferred to the medical service from the emergency room after taking a massive overdose of tricyclic antidepressants has just emerged from coma.	• Assess the patient's ongoing suicide risk, and re-evaluate the treatment strategy for his depression. Provide support and advice to family members.

C. Patients undergoing surgery

  1. Patients who are at greatest risk

   a. Those who believe that they will not survive surgery
   b. Those who do not admit that they are worried before surgery

  2. Steps to reduce psychological and medical risk

   a. Encourage the patient to take a positive attitude.
   b. Encourage the patient to talk about her fears.
   c. Explain what to expect during and after the procedure (e.g., mechanical support, pain).

D. Patients treated in the ICU or CCU

  1. Patients treated in the ICU or CCU are at increased risk for depression and delirium (ICU psychosis).

  2. Because these patients have serious, life-threatening illnesses, their clinical stability is particularly vulnerable to psychiatric symptoms.

  3. Psychological and medical risk in these patients can be reduced by **enhancing sensory input** (e.g., encouraging the patient to display personal photographs) and allowing the patient to control her environment (e.g., lighting, pain medication) as much as possible.

25

Psychopharmacology

I. ANTIPSYCHOTIC AGENTS (Table 25-1)

A. Overview

    1. Antipsychotics are pharmacologic agents that are used to treat schizophrenia (see Chapter 11) and psychotic symptoms associated with other psychiatric disorders and physical illnesses.

    2. Antipsychotic agents have a number of other clinical uses (see Table 25-1).

    3. **Drug interactions** occur between antipsychotics and central nervous system depressants, antihypertensives, anticholinergics, antidepressants, antacids, nicotine, epinephrine, propranolol, and warfarin.

B. Classification of antipsychotic agents

    1. **"Traditional"** antipsychotic agents (formerly called "neuroleptics" or "major tranquilizers") are classified according to their potency (see Table 25-1).

    2. **"Atypical"** antipsychotics work on different neurotransmitter receptors and cause different side effects than traditional agents (see Chapter 11). These agents are now used as first-line treatments because of their better side effect profiles.

II. ANTIDEPRESSANT AND MOOD-STABILIZING AGENTS

A. Overview

    1. Heterocyclic antidepressants (tricyclic and tetracyclic), monoamine oxidase inhibitors (MAOIs), selective serotonin reuptake inhibitors (SSRIs), atypical antidepressants, and sympathomimetic agents (amphetamines) are used to treat depression (Table 25-2) (see Chapter 13).

    2. With the exception of amphetamines, **antidepressants do not elevate normal mood and do not have any abuse potential.**

    3. Partly because they can be abused, amphetamines are used as antidepressants only in people who do not respond to treatment or cannot tolerate the adverse effects of other antidepressants or electroconvulsive therapy (ECT). They are used to treat depression in both the elderly and the terminally ill where abuse potential is not an issue. They are sometimes used when an immediate antidepressant effect is needed, because almost all of the other pharmacologic agents take at least several weeks to work.

    4. Lithium and thyroid hormones, particularly liothyronine (Cytomel), can be used to augment the effects of antidepressants.

Table 25-1.
Antipsychotic Medications

Type of Agent	Agent (current or former brand name)	Oral Dose (mg/day)	Special Clinical Uses in Addition to Psychotic Disorders
Traditional low-potency agents: more likely to cause anticholinergic side effects, sedation and orthostatic hypotension	Chlorpromazine (Thorazine)	100–800	Nausea and vomiting, hiccups
	Thioridazine (Mellaril)	200–600	Depression with intense anxiety or agitation
Traditional high-potency agents: more likely to cause neurologic side effects (e.g., extra-pyramidal symptoms, acute dystonia, akathisia, tardive dyskinesia); less likely to cause sedation and hypotension	Haloperidol (Haldol), haloperidol decanoate (long-acting form)	2–20	Psychosis secondary to organic syndromes; Tourette disorder and Huntington disease
	Fluphenazine (Prolixin)	2–15	Available in long-acting (decanoate) form
	Trifluoperazine (Stelazine)	4–20	Nonpsychotic anxiety (may be used for as long as 12 weeks)
	Perphenazine (Trilafon)	8–64	Nausea and vomiting
	Pimozide (Orap)	1–10	Tourette disorder, body dysmorphic disorder
Atypical agents: fewer neurologic side effects	Clozapine (Clozaril)	300–900	Negative, chronic, and refractory symptoms
	Risperidone (Risperdal)	4–16	Useful for negative symptoms: fewer hematologic problems than clozapine
	Olanzapine (Zyprexa)	10–20	
	Quetiapine (Seroquel)	50–800	
	Ziprasadone (Geodon)	40–200	
	Aripiprazole (Abilify)	10–30	

    5. Antidepressants have many **other clinical uses** in medicine and psychiatry (see Table 25-2).

  B. Heterocyclic antidepressants

    1. Heterocyclic antidepressants block the reuptake of norepinephrine and serotonin in the synapse, increase the availability of these neurotransmitters, and improve mood (see Chapter 13).

    2. The mechanism of action is not clear, but may involve post-synaptic receptor down-regulation.

    3. Because heterocyclics also block muscarinic acetylcholine and histamine receptors, they cause anticholinergic effects, sedation, and weight gain. Most are also dangerous in overdose (see Table 25-2).

Table 25-2.
Antidepressant Agents

Agent (current or former brand name)	Oral Dose (mg/day)	Effects	Special Clinical Uses in Addition to Depression
HETEROCYCLIC AGENTS (HCAs)*			
Amitriptyline (Elavil)	75–300	Sedating, anticholinergic	Depression with insomnia, chronic pain
Clomipramine (Anafranil)	100–250	Most serotonin-specific of the HCAs	Obsessive-compulsive disorder (OCD)
Desipramine (Norpramin, Pertofrane)	75–300	Least sedating, least anticholinergic, stimulates appetite	Depression in the elderly, anorexia nervosa, bulimia
Doxepin (Adapin, Sinequan)	150–300	Sedating, antihistaminic, anticholinergic	Generalized anxiety disorder, peptic ulcer disease
Imipramine (Tofranil)	150–300	Likely to cause orthostatic hypotension	Panic disorder with agoraphobia, enuresis, anorexia nervosa, bulimia
Maprotiline (Ludiomil)	150–225	Low cardiotoxicity, may cause seizures	Anxiety with depressive features
Nortriptyline (Aventyl, Pamelor)	50–150	Least likely to cause orthostatic hypotension	Depression in the elderly and patients with cardiac diseases
SELECTIVE SEROTONIN REUPTAKE INHIBITORS (SSRIs)			
Fluoxetine (Prozac, Sarafem, Prozac Weekly)	20–80 (Prozac) 20–60 (Sarafem) 90 (Prozac Weekly)	May cause agitation and insomnia initially; causes sexual dysfunction	OCD, premature ejaculation, panic disorder, pre-menstrual dysphoric disorder (Sarafem), paraphilias, hypo-chondriasis, social phobia, chronic pain, PTSD, migraine headaches, bulimia
Paroxetine [Paxil, Paxil CR (long-acting form)]	20–60	Most serotonin-specific of the SSRIs; causes sexual dysfunction	
Sertraline (Zoloft)	50–200	Most likely of the SSRIs to cause gastrointestinal disturbances (e.g., diarrhea); causes sexual dysfunction	
Fluvoxamine (Luvox)	100–300	Currently indicated only for OCD	
Citalopram (Celexa)	20–60	May be more dangerous in overdose than other SSRIs	
Escitalopram (Lexapro)	10–20	Most serotonin-specific of the SSRIs; fewer side effects than citalopram	

(continued)

Table 25-2.—*Continued*
Antidepressant Agents

Agent (current or former brand name)	Oral Dose (mg/day)	Effects	Special Clinical Uses in Addition to Depression
MONOAMINE OXIDASE INHIBITORS (MAOIs)			
Phenelzine (Nardil)	60–90	Hyperadrenergic crisis precipitated by ingestion of pressor amines in tyramine-containing foods or sympathomimetic drugs, orthostatic hypotension, sexual dysfunction, insomnia	Atypical depression, panic disorder, eating disorders, pain disorders, social phobia (phenelzine)
Tranylcypromine (Parnate)	20–60		
OTHER ANTIDEPRESSANTS			
Amoxapine (Asendin)	200–400	Antidopaminergic effects like Parkinsonian symptoms, galactorrhea, sexual dysfunction; most dangerous in overdose	Depression with psychotic features
Bupropion [Wellbutrin, Wellbutrin SR (sustained-release form), Zyban]	200–450 (Wellbutrin) 200–400 (Wellbutrin SR) 150–300 (Zyban)	Insomnia, seizures, sweating, fewer adverse sexual effects, decreased appetite	Refractory depression (inadequate clinical response to other antidepressants), smoking cessation (Zyban), seasonal affective disorder (SAD), and adult attention deficit hyperactivity disorder, SSRI-induced sexual dysfunction
Mirtazapine (Remeron)	15–45	Targets specific serotonin receptors and causes fewer sexual side effects; more sedation	Refractory depression; may increase appetite, insomnia
Nefazodone (Serzone)	300–600	Related to trazodone, but causes less sedation and priapism	Refractory depression, depression with anxiety, insomnia
Trazodone (Desyrel)	200–600	Sedation, priapism; safe in overdose	Insomnia
Venlafaxine [Effexor, Effexor XR (extended-release form)]	75–375 (Effexor) 75–225 (Effexor XR)	Serotonergic and noradrenergic, has low cytochrome P450 effects; increased diastolic blood pressure at high doses; highest remission rate, fewer sexual side effects	Refractory depression (fastest action—works within 10 days)

*Most are only available in generic form.

C. SSRIs

    1. **SSRIs selectively block the reuptake of serotonin,** but have limited effects on the norepinephrine, dopamine, histamine, and acetylcholine systems.

    2. Because of their selectivity, SSRIs cause fewer side effects and are **safer in overdose** than heterocyclics or MAO inhibitors (see Chapter 13).

    3. SSRIs have become the first-line treatment for most patients with depressive illness.

D. **MAO inhibitors**

    1. MAO inhibitors irreversibly limit the activity of monoamine oxidase, increase the availability of norepinephrine and serotonin in the synapse, and improve mood.

    2. MAO metabolizes tyramine, a pressor, in the gastrointestinal tract.

        a. If MAO is inhibited, foods that are rich in tyramine (e.g., aged cheese, chicken or beef liver, smoked or pickled meats or fish, broad beans, beer, red wine) or sympathomimetic drugs [e.g., ephedrine, methylphenidate (Ritalin), phenylephrine (Neo-Synephrine), pseudoephedrine (Sudafed)] can increase the level of **tyramine** and cause a **hypertensive crisis,** which can lead to stroke and death.

        b. MAOIs and SSRIs used together can cause another potentially life-threatening drug-drug interaction, the **serotonin syndrome,** marked by autonomic instability, hyperthermia, convulsions, coma, and death.

        c. A patient who eats in an unfamiliar place (e.g., a restaurant) may **unwittingly ingest** tyramine-containing foods.

        d. *PATIENT SNAPSHOT* A 26-year-old man who has taken phenelzine for 2 months comes to the emergency room with elevated blood pressure, sweating, headache, and vomiting. At a party he ate pizza that contained aged Parmesan cheese and drank punch that contained red wine.

E. **Mood-stabilizing agents** (Table 25-3)

    1. Lithium (carbonate and citrate), which takes 1 to 2 weeks to work, is the primary treatment to abort the manic phase of bipolar disorder.

        a. Lithium is also a mood stabilizer that is used **to prevent** both the manic and the depressive phases of bipolar disorder.

        b. Lithium is also used to **augment the effectiveness of antidepressant agents** in depressive illness.

    2. Newer anticonvulsants that may have mood-stabilizing effects include lamotrigine (Lamictal), gabapentin (Neurontin), topiramate (Topamax), and tiagabine (Gabitril).

    3. Valproic acid, divalproex, and the newer anticonvulsant agents are used to treat bipolar disorder, particularly the mixed episode (e.g., mania and depression occurring in the same episode) and rapid cycling (at least four episodes of mania and depression yearly) types.

III. ANTIANXIETY AGENTS (Table 25-4)

A. **Benzodiazepines**

    1. Benzodiazepines are used to treat anxiety and are useful also in other disorders.

    2. Their **onset of action** may be short or intermediate.

    3. Their **duration of action** may be short, intermediate, or long.

Table 25-3.
Mood Stabilizing Agents

Agent (current or former brand name)	Oral Dose (mg/day)	Adverse Effects	Special Clinical Uses in Addition to Mania
Lithium [Eskalith, Eskalith CR (controlled release)]	900–1800 (titrated to a blood level of 0.8–1.2 mEq/L), although levels of 0.6–0.8 mEq/L may be adequate	First-trimester congenital abnormalities (especially Ebstein's anomaly, a cardiac malformation), tremor, renal dysfunction, cardiac conduction problems, hypothyroidism, acne, gastric distress, mild cognitive impairment	Mood stabilization (prophylaxis for both manic and depressive episodes), control of aggressive behavior, enhancement of the activity of tricyclic antidepressants, premenstrual dysphoric disorder, borderline personality disorder, bulimia nervosa, cluster headaches
Carbamazepine (Tegretol)	400–1000 (titrated to a blood level of 4–12 μg/ml)	Aplastic anemia, agranulocytosis, sedation, dizziness, ataxia, congenital anomalies	Anticonvulsant; trigeminal neuralgia; impulse control disorders; withdrawal from sedatives
Valproic acid (Depakene) Divalproex [Depakote (more slowly absorbed form of valproic acid)]	500–1500 (titrated to a blood level of 50–100 μg/ml)	Gastrointestinal symptoms, liver problems, congenital neural tube defects, alopecia, weight gain	Anticonvulsant; migraine headaches; bipolar symptoms resulting from cognitive disorders; mixed episode and rapid cycling bipolar disorder; impulse control disorders; withdrawal from sedatives
Oxcarbazepine (Trileptal)	300–1200 (titrated to a blood level of 4–12 μg/ml)	Dizziness, ataxia, visual disturbances, no blood dyscrasias or autoinduction	Anticonvulsant, trigeminal neuralgia
Topiramate (Topamax)	400	Psychomotor slowing, fatigue	Anticonvulsant

4. Their duration of action is related to their clinical indications and their potential for abuse; for example, short-acting agents are good hypnotics (sleep inducers) and also have a higher potential for abuse.

B. **Nonbenzodiazepines**

1. The azapirone buspirone (BuSpar) is unrelated to the benzodiazepines. Its advantages are that it is nonsedating and is not associated with dependence, abuse, or withdrawal. However, it takes a few weeks to work and is often ineffective, particularly in patients who have abused alcohol or benzodiazepines.

Table 25-4.

Antianxiety Agents (in order of duration of action by category)

Agent (brand name or former brand name)	Oral Dose (mg/day)	Onset of Action	Duration of Action	Special Clinical Uses in Addition to Anxiety
BENZODIAZEPINES				
Clorazepate (Tranxene)	15–60	Short	Short	Adjunctive use in the management of partial seizures
Alprazolam (Xanax)	0.5–10	Short	Short	Antidepressant; panic disorder; social phobia
Oxazepam (Serax)	30–120	Intermediate	Short	Alcohol withdrawal
Triazolam (Halcion)	0.125–0.50	Intermediate	Short	Insomnia
Lorazepam (Ativan)	2–10	Intermediate	Intermediate	Psychotic agitation, alcohol withdrawal, status epilepticus
Temazepam (Restoril)	15–30	Intermediate	Intermediate	Insomnia
Chlordiazepoxide (Librium)	15–100	Short	Long	Alcohol withdrawal
Clonazepam (Klonopin)	0.5–4	Short	Long	Seizures, mania, social phobia, panic disorder, aggression, adjunctive use with mood stabilizers
Diazepam (Valium)	4–40	Short	Long	Muscle relaxation, analgesia, anticonvulsant
Flurazepam (Dalmane)	15–30	Short	Long	Insomnia
NONBENZODIAZEPINES				
Zolpidem (Ambien)	5–10	Short	Short	Insomnia
Zaleplon (Sonata)	10–20	Short	Short	Insomnia
Buspirone (BuSpar)	15–60	Very long	Very long	Anxiety in the elderly; low abuse potential; no sedation

2. Zolpidem tartrate (Ambien) and zaleplon (Sonata) are hypnotics that are unrelated to the benzodiazepines.

3. Carbamates (e.g., meprobamate; Miltown) have a greater potential for abuse and a lower therapeutic index than benzodiazepines. They are used only rarely now, and are largely of historical interest.

4. Antihypertensive agents, including the β-antagonists (β-blockers) such as propranolol (Inderal) and α_2 adrenergic receptor antagonists such as clonidine (Catapres), serve to decrease the autonomic hyperarousal associated with somatic anxiety and with withdrawal from opiates and sedatives.

IV. ELECTROCONVUSIVE THERAPY (ECT)

A. Uses

1. ECT involves inducing a generalized seizure lasting 25 to 60 seconds by passing an electric current through the brain in one of three ways: bilateral ECT (one electrode placed on each temple), bifrontal ECT (one electrode placed above the end of each eyebrow), and unilateral ECT (two electrodes placed on the nondominant hemisphere). ECT is a safe, effective treatment for **major depressive disorder refractive to other treatment,** the most common indication. It is more effective for depression with psychotic features than antidepressants or antipsychotics administered alone or both types given concurrently. It is also effective for treatment of acute mania and schizophrenia with acute, catatonic, or affective symptoms.

2. The maximum response to ECT usually occurs after **5 to 10 treatments given over a 2 to 3 week period.** Biweekly or monthly maintenance ECT may be used to prevent relapse.

B. Adverse effects

1. Most adverse affects, such as broken bones, have been eliminated with judicious use of general anesthesia [e.g., methohexital (Brevital)] and muscle relaxants [e.g., succinylcholine (Anectine)] before treatment. The mortality rate is comparable to that associated with general anesthesia.

2. The major adverse effect of ECT is amnesia for past events. In most patients, amnesia resolves within 6 months after treatment concludes.

3. ECT is contraindicated in patients with increased intracranial pressure from any cause or recent (within two weeks) myocardial infarction.

4. Unilateral and bifrontal electrode placement cause less memory impairment but slower therapeutic responses than bilateral electrode placement.

26

Psychoanalysis and Related Therapies

I. FREUDIAN THEORY

A. Overview

    1. Psychoanalysis and related therapies are based on Freud's idea that behavior is determined (**psychic determinism or psychic causality**) by forces derived from **unconscious mental processes.**

    2. Psychoanalysis and related psychotherapies include:

        a. Classic psychoanalysis
        b. Psychoanalytically oriented psychotherapy
        c. Brief dynamic therapy
        d. Interpersonal therapy

B. **Theories of the mind.** Freud's early (topographic) and later (structural) theories of the mind were developed to explain his ideas (Table 26-1).

II. DEFENSE MECHANISMS

A. Overview

    1. Defense mechanisms are **unconscious** mental techniques used by the ego to keep conflicts out of awareness, reduce anxiety, and maintain a person's self-esteem and sense of safety and equilibrium. The mechanisms are enacted by the "ego" component of the mind (see Table 26-1).

    2. The fundamental defense mechanism is **repression.**

        a. In repression, the patient pushes unacceptable feelings into the unconscious (e.g., a man does not remember that he was sexually abused as a child).
        b. All other defense mechanisms are based on repression.

    3. Although defense mechanisms protect the organism, if any one is used exclusively or excessively, neurotic symptoms will result.

    4. Altruism, humor, sublimation, and suppression are **"mature"** defense mechanisms because, when used in moderation, they directly help the patient or others.

    5. Denial, projection, and splitting are often pathological defense mechanisms.

B. Specific defense mechanisms are shown in Table 26-2.

III. PSYCHOANALYSIS

A. The central strategy of psychoanalysis is to slowly uncover experiences that are repressed in the unconscious mind and then integrate them into the patient's personality.

Table 26-1.
Freud's Topographic and Structural Theories of the Mind

Theory	Component of the Mind	Characteristics and Functions
Topographic	Unconscious	Contains repressed thoughts and feelings; uses **primary process** thinking (e.g., has no logic or concept of time, and involves primitive drives, wish fulfillment, and pleasure seeking); primary process is also common in young children and psychotic adults
	Preconscious	Contains memories that are not immediately available, but can be retrieved readily and brought to consciousness.
	Conscious	The thoughts that an individual is currently aware of. Operates in conjunction with the preconscious, but cannot access the unconscious directly. Uses **secondary process** thinking (e.g., logical, time-oriented, mature, delays gratification)
Structural	Id	Present at birth and controlled by primary process thinking; contains instinctual sexual and aggressive drives; acts in concert with the pleasure principle and is not influenced by external reality; operates almost completely on an unconscious level
	Ego	Begins to develop immediately after birth; controls the expression of instinctual drives, primarily by the use of defense mechanisms to adapt to the requirements of the external world; maintains a relationship with the external world; evaluates what is valid (i.e., reality testing), adapts to that reality, and maintains satisfying interpersonal or object relations; operates on unconscious, preconscious, and conscious levels
	Superego	Developed by approximately 6 years of age; associated with conscience and morality; operates on unconscious, preconscious, and conscious levels

B. Techniques that are used to recover repressed experiences include:

1. Free association (i.e., the patient lies on a couch in a reclined position facing away from the therapist and says whatever comes to mind). Layer by layer, unconscious memories are revealed, and the therapist interprets the information.

2. Interpretation of dreams as representations of conflict between fears and wishes (satisfaction of unconscious instinctual impulses)

3. Analysis of transference reactions (i.e., the patient's reactions to the therapist) to examine important past relationships

4. Analysis of resistance (i.e., blocking unconscious thoughts from consciousness because the patient finds them unacceptable)

C. Patients who are **appropriate for psychoanalysis:**

1. Are younger than 40 years of age

2. Are intelligent

3. Are not psychotic

4. Have good relationships with others (e.g., no evidence of antisocial or borderline personality disorder)

5. Have a stable life situation

6. Can spend considerable time and money on treatment

Table 26-2.
Specific Defense Mechanisms (in Alphabetical Order)

Defense Mechanism	Definition	Patient Snapshot
Acting out	Avoiding unacceptable emotions by behaving in an attention-getting, often socially inappropriate manner	A depressed 15-year-old boy with no history of conduct disorder steals a car after his parents separate.
Altruism	Assisting others in order to avoid negative personal feelings	A man with a poor self-image gives one-fifth of his annual salary to charity.
Denial	Not accepting aspects of reality that the individual finds unbearable	An active 54-year-old woman insists that a laboratory report that shows that she has had a myocardial infarction is in error.
Displacement	Moving emotions from a personally unacceptable situation to one that is personally tolerable	A surgical resident with unacknowledged anger toward her husband is abrasive to the male medical students on her service.
Dissociation	Mentally separating part of one's consciousness or mentally distancing oneself from others	A soldier has no memory of a battle in which his best friend was killed.
Humor	Expressing feelings without causing discomfort	A man who is uncomfortable with his pattern baldness makes jokes about hair restoration techniques.
Identification (with the aggressor)	Patterning one's behavior after that of someone more powerful (may be positive or negative)	A man who was physically abused in childhood by his father abuses his own children.
Intellectualization	Using the mind's higher functions to avoid experiencing emotion; associated with obsessive-compulsive personality disorder	In normal conversation with colleagues, a physician explains the technical details of the treatment options for his own terminal illness.
Isolation of affect	Failing to experience the feelings associated with a stressful life event, although the person logically understands the significance of the event	Although he was close to her, a man whose mother recently died describes the circumstances of her death dispassionately.
Projection	Attributing one's unacceptable feelings to others; associated with paranoid symptoms and ordinary prejudice	A woman who has unacknowledged and unacceptable feelings for other men believes (without evidence) that her husband is cheating on her.
Rationalization	Distorting one's perception of an event so that its negative outcome seems reasonable	A job candidate who is not hired says, "I'm glad. That was a dead-end job anyway."

(continued)

Table 26-2.—*Continued*

Specific Defense Mechanisms (in Alphabetical Order)

Defense Mechanism	Definition		Patient Snapshot
Reaction formation	Adopting opposite attitudes to avoid unacceptable emotions; unlike hypocrisy, this is an unconscious process		A man who is angry with his physician compliments her clothing.
Regression	Reverting to behavior patterns typical of a younger person; seen in patients with dependent personality disorder		A woman who is hospitalized for minor surgery insists that her husband not leave her room.
Splitting	Categorizing people (or even the same person at different times) as either "perfect" or "awful"; intolerance of ambiguity; seen in patients with borderline personality disorder		A hospitalized patient says that all of the weekday doctors are cold and insensitive, but that the weekend doctors are warm and friendly.
Sublimation	Expressing an unacceptable impulse in a socially useful way		A medical student with strong destructive impulses chooses to do a residency in surgery.
Suppression	Deliberately pushing unacceptable emotions out of conscious awareness		An emergency room resident chooses to put aside his feelings of disgust and pity so that he can deal with the medical needs of the victims of a fire.
Undoing	Believing that one can magically reverse events caused by "wrong" behavior by adopting "right" behavior		A woman who is diagnosed with terminal lung cancer as a result of smoking buys books on nutrition, stops smoking, and starts to exercise.

D. Patients receive treatment four to five times weekly for 3–4 years.

E. Transference and countertransference are phenomena that occur during psychoanalysis as well as in ordinary physician–patient relationships (Table 26-3).

IV. RELATED THERAPIES

A. Psychoanalytically oriented psychotherapy (including brief dynamic psychotherapy)

    1. Similarities to psychoanalysis

        a. They are **insight-oriented** (i.e., aim to understand the underlying unconscious basis for current conflicts and behaviors).

        b. They may use dream interpretation and analysis of transference reactions.

    2. Differences from psychoanalysis

        a. They are **briefer and more direct** (e.g., brief dynamic psychotherapy is limited to 12–40 weekly sessions).

Table 26-3.

Transference and Countertransference

Phenomenon	Definition	Patient Snapshot
Transference	Unconscious reexperiencing of feelings about parents or important figures in the **patient's** life in his current relationship with the therapist	A 30-year-old man with a mother who often disappointed him becomes angry when his physician attempts to terminate his consultation with her.
Countertransference	Unconscious reexperiencing of feelings about parents or other important figures in the **therapist's** life in her current relationship with the patient	A physician becomes angry with a noncompliant patient who reminds her of her obstinate son.

    b. Rather than lying on a couch and using free association, the patient sits in a chair and talks directly with the therapist.

  3. Patients who are appropriate for psychoanalytically oriented psychotherapy:

    a. Are flexible and intelligent

    b. Can tolerate the emotions that may surface (e.g., anger, guilt)

    c. Can maintain a relationship with a therapist

    d. Are motivated to gain insight and understanding, not only to relieve symptoms

B. Interpersonal therapy and supportive psychotherapy

  1. Interpersonal therapy is based on the idea that psychiatric problems (e.g., anxiety) are caused by difficulties with interpersonal skills. It focuses on developing these skills in 12–16 weekly sessions.

  2. Supportive psychotherapy does not seek insight, but is designed to **help people feel protected** during a life crisis. All patients can benefit from support and reassurance, including psychologically well-adjusted individuals, as well as patients with mild, moderate, and severe mental disorders. Patients who are chronically mentally ill may receive supportive psychotherapy in conjunction with medication for many years.

27

Behavioral and Cognitive Therapies

I. OVERVIEW

A. Behavioral and cognitive therapies are based on **learning theory** (i.e., relieving the patient's symptoms by altering behavior and thinking patterns).

B. In contrast to psychoanalysis and related therapies, the patient's history and unconscious conflicts are not explored because they are considered irrelevant.

II. CHARACTERISTICS OF SPECIFIC THERAPIES (Table 27-1)

Table 27-1.
Behavioral and Cognitive Therapies: Uses, Strategies, and Patient Snapshots

Specific Therapy	Most Common Use	Strategy		Patient Snapshot
Systemic desensitization	Treatment of phobias (irrational fears; see Chapter 14)	Through the process of classical conditioning, the patient, some time in the past, began to associate an innocuous object with a fear-provoking object, until the innocuous thing became frightening. Here, increasing doses of the frightening stimulus are paired with a relaxing stimulus to provoke a relaxation response. Because one cannot simultaneously be fearful and relaxed (reciprocal inhibition), the patient shows less anxiety when exposed to the frightening stimulus in the future.	PATIENT SNAPSHOT	A 38-year-old woman who is afraid to fly is taught relaxation techniques and is then shown a photograph of an airplane. Later in treatment, she is exposed to toy planes, then to real planes on the ground. Finally, she takes a plane ride.

(continued)

Table 27-1.—*Continued*

Behavioral and Cognitive Therapies: Uses, Strategies, and Patient Snapshots

Specific Therapy	Most Common Use	Strategy		Patient Snapshot
Aversive conditioning	Treatment of paraphilias or addictions (e.g., drinking, smoking)	Classical conditioning is used to pair a maladaptive but pleasurable stimulus with an aversive or painful stimulus (e.g., a shock) so that the two become associated. The patient ultimately stops engaging in the maladaptive behavior, because it automatically provokes an unpleasant response.	*PATIENT SNAPSHOT*	A 35-year-old man with pedophilia is given an electric shock each time he is shown a videotape of children. Later, he feels uncomfortable around children, and avoids them.
Flooding and implosion	Treatment of phobias	Through the process of habituation, the patient is exposed to an actual (flooding) or imagined (implosion) overwhelming dose of the feared object until she becomes accustomed to it and is no longer afraid.	*PATIENT SNAPSHOT*	• A woman who is afraid of airplanes agrees to take a 14-hour flight to Australia (flooding). • A woman who is afraid of airplanes agrees to imagine being on a plane that is leaving on a 14-hour flight to Australia (implosion).
Token economy	To increase positive behavior in a person who is mentally retarded or severely disorganized	Through the process of operant conditioning, desirable behavior (e.g., shaving, hair combing) is differentially reinforced by a reward or positive reinforcement (e.g., the token)	*PATIENT SNAPSHOT*	A 23-year-old man who is mentally retarded is given a token each time he shaves. He can exchange tokens for treats at the hospital store. He begins to shave every day.
Biofeedback	To treat hypertension, migraine and tension headaches, asthma, Raynaud disease, chronic pain, fecal incontinence, and temporomandibular joint pain	Through the process of operant conditioning, the patient is given ongoing physiologic information (e.g., blood pressure measurement). The patient uses this information to control visceral changes (e.g., heart rate, blood pressure, smooth muscle tone)	*PATIENT SNAPSHOT*	A 50-year-old man with hypertension has his blood pressure measured regularly. The readings are projected to him on a computer screen. He is then taught to use mental techniques to decrease his blood pressure.

(*continued*)

Table 27-1.—*Continued*
Behavioral and Cognitive Therapies: Uses, Strategies, and Patient Snapshots

Specific Therapy	Most Common Use	Strategy		Patient Snapshot
Cognitive therapy	To treat mild-to-moderate depression, somatoform disorders, eating disorders	Weekly, for as long as 25 weeks, the patient is helped to identify distorted, negative thoughts about herself and replace them with positive, self-assuring thoughts.		A 38-year-old woman with depression is told to replace each self-deprecating thought with a mental image of success and praise.

28

Group, Family, and Marital Therapy

I. GROUP THERAPY

A. A 35-year-old woman joins a therapy group that consists of women who have been abused by their partners. The group is led by a psychotherapist who is trained in domestic violence issues.

B. Primary uses

 1. People with a **common problem** (e.g., substance abusers, rape victims)

 2. People with **personality disorders** or other interpersonal problems

 3. People who have **trouble interacting with authority figures** (e.g., those who cannot deal with therapists in individual therapy)

C. Characteristics

 1. Groups usually meet weekly for 1–2 hours.

 2. The optimal number of people in a group is 6–10.

 3. Members of the group provide feedback, support, friendship, and the opportunity to express feelings.

 4. The therapist facilitates and observes the patients' interpersonal interactions, but has little input.

D. Leaderless groups

 1. A leaderless group has no one person (e.g., therapist) in authority.

 2. Members of the group **share a problem** (e.g., alcoholism, loss of a loved one, a specific illness) and provide each other with support, friendship, acceptance, and the opportunity to express feelings.

 3. **Twelve-step** peer support groups like Narcotics Anonymous (NA) and Overeaters Anonymous (OA) are based on the Alcoholics Anonymous (AA) model (see Chapter 10).

II. FAMILY THERAPY

A. A 12-year-old boy who is argumentative, angry, and resentful toward adults (oppositional defiant disorder; see Chapter 4), his parents, and his sister meet with a therapist for 2 hours each week.

B. Primary uses

 1. Behavioral problems in children

2. Family conflict

3. Eating disorders

4. Substance abuse

C. Family systems theory

1. Family therapy is based on the idea that psychopathology in one family member (i.e., the identified patient) reflects dysfunction of the entire family system.

2. Because all members of the family cause reactions in other members, the family, rather than the identified patient, is really the patient **(circular causality rather than linear causality).**

D. Strategy of family therapy

1. Identifying dyads, triangles, and boundaries

   a. Dyads are subsystems between two family members (e.g., the "executive subsystem" normally contains the two parents).
   b. Boundaries are barriers between subsystems (e.g., between the executive subsystem and the children). They may be too rigid or too permeable.
   c. Triangles are dysfunctional alliances between two family members against a third member (e.g., the father and daughter against the mother).

2. Techniques used in family therapy

   a. Encouraging **"mutual accommodation,"** a process in which family members identify each other's needs and work toward meeting them
   b. Normalizing boundaries between subsystems and reducing the likelihood of triangles
   c. Redefining "blame" and encouraging family members to reconsider their own responsibility for problems

III. MARITAL THERAPY

A. A man and a woman who have been married for 8 years and have two children argue constantly and are considering divorce because the husband confessed to an affair.

B. Primary uses. To explore and resolve:

1. Communication problems

2. Psychosexual problems

3. Differences in values

C. Types

1. Conjoint therapy. One therapist sees the couple together (most common type).

2. Concurrent therapy. One therapist sees both members of the couple individually.

3. Collaborative therapy. Two therapists (usually one for each member of the couple) see both members of the couple individually.

4. Four-way therapy. Two therapists (one for each member of the couple) see the couple together; used most commonly for sexual problems.

29
Legal Issues in Psychiatry and Medicine

I. ADVANCE DIRECTIVES

A. Overview

   1. Advance directives are instructions given in anticipation of the need for a medical decision. A **living will** and a **durable power of attorney** are examples of advance directives (Table 29-1).

   2. Hospitals and nursing homes that receive Medicare payments (most institutions do) are required to ask patients whether they have advance directives and, if necessary, help patients to write them. They must also inform patients of their right to refuse treatment or resuscitation.

B. Special situations

   1. If an incompetent patient has no advance directive, health care providers or family members (surrogates) must determine what the patient would have done if she were competent (the **substituted judgment standard**), or what a reasonable person would do after weighing each course of action (the **best interest standard**). The personal wishes of surrogates are irrelevant to the medical decision.

   2. If the patient regains function (competence), even briefly or intermittently, during those periods of competence he regains the right to make decisions about his health care.

II. DEFINITION OF DEATH

A. Legal standard of death

   1. In the United States, the legal standard of death when the heart is still beating is **irreversible cessation of all functions of the entire brain including the brain stem.**

   2. A 20-year-old woman sustained brain damage after a suicide attempt. She is in a coma and requires life support. Clinical examination and EEG reveal irreversible cessation of brain function. Her father instructs the physician not to withdraw life support.

   3. If the patient is legally dead ("brain dead"), the physician is authorized to remove life support without a court order. The father's request is not relevant to this decision.

B. Role of the physician

   1. Certify the cause of death (e.g., natural, suicide, accident).

   2. Sign the death certificate.

Table 29-1.
Advance Directives: Living Will and Durable Power of Attorney

Advance Directive	Definition		Patient Snapshot	Appropriate Action
Living will	A document in which a patient gives directions for his future health care if he becomes incompetent to make decisions when he needs care	PATIENT SNAPSHOT	A 65-year-old man signs a document that states that he does not want heroic measures taken to save his life if he enters a persistent vegetative state. Five days later, he has a stroke, goes into a coma, and has no realistic chance of regaining consciousness. His wife urges the physician to save her husband's life.	The physician should take heroic measures only if he expects the patient to recover. This decision is medical and is based on the patient's instructions; the wife's wishes are not relevant.
Durable power of attorney	A document in which a patient designates another person (e.g., her husband) as her legal representative to make decisions about her health care when she can no longer do so	PATIENT SNAPSHOT	A 65-year-old woman signs a document that gives her husband durable power of attorney. Five days later, she has a stroke, goes into a coma, and enters a persistent vegetative state.	The husband can decide whether to continue life support. Essentially, the husband has assumed the power to speak for the patient by virtue of the document.

   3. **Provide support** and counseling to family members.

   4. When appropriate, request permission to perform an **autopsy.**

C. Euthanasia

   1. According to medical codes of ethics (e.g., American Medical Association, medical specialty organizations), **active euthanasia is a criminal act** and is **never appropriate.**

   2. Physician-assisted suicide (e.g., Dr. Kevorkian cases) is not strictly legal in any state, but is not generally an indictable offense as long as the physician does not actually perform the killing (i.e., active euthanasia).

   3. Under most circumstances, food, water, medical care, and artificial life support can be withheld from a comatose terminally ill patient who has no reasonable prospect of recovery, although not legally dead (i.e., passive euthanasia).

III. THE RIGHT TO DIE AND RELATED ISSUES

   A. Refusal of treatment

1. A 30-year-old man and his 10-year-old son are injured in a train crash. Both of them need surgery. The father is lucid and refuses the surgery for both himself and his son because of religious reasons.

2. A patient who is competent (see III B) can refuse lifesaving treatment **for himself** for religious or other reasons, even if death will be the outcome.

3. A parent cannot refuse lifesaving treatment **for his minor child** for any reason. In a nonemergency situation, a court order must be obtained before treatment can be started. In an emergency, the physician can proceed without a court order.

4. A competent pregnant woman can refuse treatment (e.g., cesarean section) that is intended **to save the life of her fetus,** even if the fetus will die or be seriously injured without the treatment.

5. It is both legal and ethical for a physician to halt artificial life support systems if requested to do so by a competent patient.

B. Legal issues

1. To be legally **competent** to accept or refuse medical treatment, the patient must understand:

   a. The risks and benefits of the treatment
   b. The likely outcome if the treatment is refused

2. If a person's competence is in question, a **judge** (not the patient's family or physician) makes the determination of competence.

3. **Minors** (people younger than 18 years of age) usually are not considered competent unless they meet certain criteria to accept or refuse medical treatment ("emancipated minors," see Chapter 30).

4. A person may still meet the legal standard for competence to accept or refuse medical treatment even if she is **mentally ill or retarded** or is incompetent in other areas of her life (e.g., with finances).

IV. INVOLUNTARY HOSPITALIZATION OF PATIENTS WITH PSYCHIATRIC DISORDERS

A. Under certain circumstances that vary according to state law (Table 29-2), patients with psychiatric disorders may be hospitalized against their will. For involuntary hospitalization, a patient usually must be dangerous to self or others or unable to provide self-care (not merely self-neglect).

B. The Mental Health Bill of Rights may vary in details from state to state. In general, a patient who is confined to a mental health facility, either voluntarily or involuntarily, has the following rights:

1. The right to **receive appropriate treatment**

2. The right to **refuse treatment** (e.g., medication, electroconvulsive therapy (ECT), surgical procedures). However, in some cases, medication or ECT may be administered against the patient's wishes to prevent danger to the patient or to others.

3. The right to **privacy**

4. The right to **manage his own finances,** unless he is declared legally incompetent

5. The right to receive **visitors**

6. The right to **communicate** with the outside world

7. The right to receive **payment for work** he performs in the facility

Table 29-2.

Voluntary, Emergency, and Involuntary Hospitalization of Patients With Psychiatric Disorders

Patient Snapshot	Intervention	Comment
A 45-year-old man with paranoid schizophrenia who lives in a subway station is brought to the emergency room. He is dirty and malnourished, and refuses to be hospitalized.	No intervention	The patient cannot be involuntarily hospitalized because he does not pose a significant danger to himself or to others. Self-neglect is not grounds for involuntary hospitalization unless it constitutes a significant, imminent danger to his life.
A 45-year-old man with paranoid schizophrenia who lives in a subway station comes to the emergency room and asks to be hospitalized. After 4 hours, he demands to be released.	Voluntary hospitalization	Voluntary hospitalization is used for patients who choose to be hospitalized; however, unlike most medical admissions, patients who have psychiatric disorders and are voluntarily hospitalized may be required to wait 24–48 hours before they are permitted to sign out against medical advice.
A 45-year-old man with paranoid schizophrenia who lives in a subway station is brought to the emergency room because he tried to jump onto the tracks just as a train was coming. He refuses hospitalization.	Emergency or involuntary hospitalization	Emergency or involuntary hospitalization is used for patients who will not or cannot agree to be hospitalized; it requires the certification of one physician (emergency hospitalization: "one-physician certificate") or two physicians (involuntary hospitalization: "two-physician certificate"). The patient can be held for as long as 15 days (emergency hospitalization) or 60 days (involuntary hospitalization), before a court hearing, depending on state laws. The court may repeatedly extend the confinement for 3 months or more at a time.

V. CRIMINAL LAW

A. Intent

1. A 22-year-old woman who showed no previous psychiatric illness is arrested for murdering her 3-week-old son. The woman claims that God told her to kill the child (a "command" hallucination).

2. Although she committed an illegal act (i.e., homicide), the act alone is not necessarily a crime.

3. A crime requires both **evil intent** (mens rea) and an **evil deed** (actus reus). For example, a judge or jury may determine that because of her mental state (e.g., brief psychotic disorder with postpartum onset; see Chapter 12), the woman lacked the requisite state of mind to commit a crime.

B. Competence to stand trial

1. **All adults** (people 18 years of age and older), even people who are mentally ill or retarded, **are presumed to be competent** to stand trial.

2. An adult is considered unfit to stand trial (legally incompetent) if she does not understand the charges against her or cannot cooperate with counsel in the preparation of her defense.

C. Legal insanity

1. A person who is found legally insane must both have a **mental illness** and, as a result, meet one of the **statutory criteria** (Table 29-3) under state or federal law.

2. Some states and federal jurisdictions have a different set of standards (often more liberal) under which an individual with mental illness can qualify for **diminished capacity,** which may reduce the level of the crime or modify the punishment.

VI. MEDICAL MALPRACTICE

A. Overview

1. Medical malpractice occurs when a physician causes harm to a patient by deviating from an accepted standard of practice.

2. **Surgeons** (including obstetricians) and anesthesiologists are the specialists **most likely to be sued** for malpractice. **Psychiatrists** and **family practitioners** are the **least likely** to be sued.

Table 29-3.
Statutory Criteria for Legal Insanity as a Result of Mental Illness

Test	Definition	Comments
M'Naghten	Determines whether the person understands the nature and quality of his actions, and if so, whether he knows that the actions were wrong	The strictest test, and the standard criterion in most jurisdictions
American Law Institute (ALI) Model Penal Code	• Cognitive prong—determines whether the person appreciates the wrongfulness of his behavior. • Volitional prong—determines whether the person is able to conform his conduct to the requirements of the law	After the John Hinckley case, most jurisdictions that used this test dropped the volitional prong.
Durham	Evaluates whether the person's criminal behavior is the "product" of a mental illness	The most lenient test, it has been abandoned in almost all jurisdictions

B. The **four "Ds" of malpractice** are **dereliction,** or negligence (e.g., deviation from normal standards of care), of a **duty** (i.e., there is an established physician–patient relationship) that causes **damages** (i.e., injury) **directly** to the patient (also known as "proximate cause," meaning that the damages were caused by the negligence, not by another factor).

   1. A 45-year-old man undergoes surgery to repair a torn rotator cuff. After the surgery, the patient has partial paralysis of the affected arm and sues the surgeon for malpractice.

   2. The lawsuit will be successful if the patient can prove that the physician committed the **four Ds of malpractice.** An unfavorable outcome alone (e.g., partial paralysis of the arm as an unavoidable complication of the surgical procedure) does not constitute malpractice.

C. Sequelae of malpractice suits

   1. Malpractice is a **tort, or civil wrong,** not a crime. A finding for the plaintiff (the patient) results in a financial award (damages) to the patient from the defendant physician or his insurance carrier, not a jail term or loss of license, although the doctor's name may be listed in the National Practitioner Data Bank.

   2. The patient may be awarded compensatory damages only, or both compensatory and punitive damages.

      a. **Compensatory damages** are given to the patient to reimburse him for medical bills or lost salary (economic damages), and to compensate him for pain and suffering (noneconomic damages).

      b. **Punitive (or exemplary) damages** are awarded to the patient to punish the physician and set an example for the medical community. Punitive damages are rare and are awarded only in cases of wanton carelessness or gross negligence (e.g., a drunk surgeon cuts a vital artery).

D. Sexual relationships with patients

   1. Sexual relationships with current or former patients are **inappropriate** and are proscribed by the ethical standards of most specialty boards.

   2. A **time limit** may apply to the definition of a former patient (usually much longer for patients of psychiatrists).

   3. Patients who claim that they had a sexual relationship with a physician may file an ethics complaint or a medical malpractice complaint, or both.

   4. Many malpractice insurance carriers do not pay judgments based on improper sexual behavior, even if they agree to pay for the physician's legal defense.

E. Reasons for the recent increase in the number of malpractice claims

   1. General **increase in lawsuits**

   2. Patients' **heightened expectations** of physicians

   3. **Breakdown of the traditional physician–patient relationship** because of:

      a. Technological advances in medicine, which reduce personal contact with the doctor

      b. Limits on physician autonomy and time for personal interaction, partly as a result of the growth of managed care

30

Ethical Issues in Psychiatry and Medicine

I. CONFIDENTIALITY

A. A patient says that he plans to kill his wife as soon as he leaves the hospital. Are you required to keep this information confidential? If not, whom do you notify?

B. Although physicians are **expected ethically to maintain patient confidentiality,** they are not required to do so if the patient is placing himself or others at serious risk. Examples include:

    1. Likely **suicide attempt**

    2. Suspected **child or elder abuse**

    3. **Serious threat** to another person

C. Intervention

    1. **Determine the credibility** of the danger or threat.

    2. If the threat is credible, take one of the following appropriate actions **(the Tarasoff decision).**

        a. **Notify** the appropriate **law enforcement** officials or social service agency.
        b. Arrange to commit the patient (see Chapter 29).
        c. Warn the intended victim.

II. REPORTABLE ILLNESSES

A. A 34-year-old woman has genital herpes. Must you report the case, and if so, to whom?

B. Sexually transmitted diseases (STDs)

    1. Physicians document "reportable" illnesses to their **state health departments;** states may differ in which illnesses are reportable.

    2. State health departments report these illness (without patient names) to the federal Centers for Disease Control and Prevention (CDC) for statistical purposes.

    3. Acquired immune deficiency syndrome **(AIDS)** [but not HIV-positive status in some states] and some STDs, including **syphilis, gonorrhea,** and **chlamydia** are reportable.

    4. Genital herpes usually does not have to be reported.

C. Other reportable illnesses. In addition to STDs, most states require physicians to report infectious diseases like varicella, hepatitis, measles, mumps, rubella, salmonellosis, shigellosis, and tuberculosis.

III. IMPAIRED PHYSICIANS

A. Causes of impairment in physicians

1. Drug or alcohol abuse

2. Physical or mental illness

3. Impairment in functioning associated with old age

B. On your pediatrics rotation, you frequently smell alcohol on the breath of another medical student. You talk to him, but he denies having a drinking problem. What do you do?

C. Intervention

1. Reporting of an impaired colleague is **required ethically** because patients must be protected and the impaired colleague must be helped. The legal requirement for reporting impaired colleagues varies by state.

2. An impaired medical student should be reported to the **dean of the medical school** or the **dean of students.**

3. An impaired resident or attending physician should be reported to the **residency training director** or the **chief of the medical staff**, respectively.

4. A licensed physician should report an impaired colleague to the state licensing board or the **impaired physicians' program,** usually part of the state medical society.

IV. INFORMED CONSENT

A. Treatment of adults

1. A 60-year-old woman who has been depressed over her husband's death has a breast biopsy for a suspicious mass. Her son instructs you not to tell her the diagnosis if the results show a malignancy because he fears that she will kill herself. If the mass proves to be malignant, should you tell her?

a. Ordinarily, you must provide the patient with full information about her diagnosis before you can obtain informed consent for treatment.

b. If you believe that the patient's life or health will be adversely affected, you can delay telling her until the potential for adverse effects is reduced. The opinions of family members are not considered legally relevant, however.

c. At the patient's request, family members may be present when you give the patient her diagnosis.

2. The physician must obtain consent before any medical or surgical procedure or treatment, except for a life-threatening emergency. Other hospital personnel (e.g., nurses) usually cannot obtain informed consent.

3. Before she can give informed consent, the patient must understand:

a. The **diagnosis** or the medical finding

b. The **treatment, alternatives to treatment,** and the **risks and benefits** of treatment

c. The likely outcome if she does not consent to the procedure

d. That she can **withdraw consent** at any time before the procedure (even on the way to the operating room after preanesthetic medication has been administered)

4. Although a signature may not be required for minor medical procedures, the patient should sign a document of agreement for major medical procedures or for surgery.

5. If an **unexpected finding during surgery** necessitates a non-emergency procedure for which the patient has not given consent (e.g., biopsy of an unsuspected ovarian malignancy during a tubal ligation), the patient must wake up and give informed consent before the additional procedure can be performed.

B. Treatment of minors [i.e., people **younger than 18 years of age,** unless emancipated (see IV B 7)]

1. A 9-year-old girl is injured during gym class and has a laceration that requires stitches. Her parents cannot be located. Can the teacher or school principal give consent for her treatment?

2. Only the **parent or legal guardian** can give consent for surgical or medical treatment of a minor.

3. In an emergency, if the parent or guardian **cannot be located,** surgical or medical treatment may proceed without consent. Some schools ask parents to sign a blanket consent form at the start of the school year, but these forms have questionable legal validity.

4. A **court order** can be obtained if a child has a life-threatening illness or accident and the parent or guardian **refuses to consent to established medical treatment** for religious or other reasons (see Chapter 29).

   a. A court order can usually be obtained within hours if necessary.
   b. Courts usually do not order experimental or nonestablished procedures for children.

5. **Parental consent is not required:**

   a. In **emergency situations**
   b. For the treatment of **STDs**
   c. For prescription of **contraceptives**
   d. For medical care during **pregnancy**
   e. For the treatment of **drug and alcohol dependence**

6. Most states require parental consent when a minor seeks an abortion.

7. Minors are considered **emancipated** and can give consent for their own medical care if they meet any of the following criteria:

   a. They are **self-supporting** or in the **military.**
   b. They are **married.**
   c. They have **children** whom they care for.

V. ETHICAL ISSUES IN THE TREATMENT OF PATIENTS WITH AIDS. Table 30-1

describes ethical problems faced by physicians who treat patients with AIDS.

Table 30-1.

Ethical Issues Concerning Patients With Acquired Immune Deficiency Syndrome (AIDS)

Category and Patient Snapshot	Ethical Issue	Appropriate Action
HIV-positive patients A 25-year-old man who is HIV positive comes to a doctor's office for treatment.	Can the doctor refuse to treat him because he poses a risk to her?	No. The doctor may not refuse to treat him for this reason.
HIV-exposed physicians A 40-year-old female physician is stuck with a needle that she had just used to draw blood from a patient with AIDS.	Must the physician be tested for HIV?	For medical and ethical reasons, the physician should be tested, but it is not legally required.
HIV-positive colleagues A colleague to whom you have regularly referred patients tells you that he is HIV positive.	Should you continue to refer your patients to him, and should you tell the patients about his HIV status?	Yes, you should continue to refer patients provided that: (1) he is physically and mentally competent to treat them and (2) he complies with precautions for infection control. You are not required to inform either patients or the medical establishment about his HIV-positive status.
HIV-positive patients who put others at risk A 30-year-old man who is HIV positive tells you that he is having unprotected sex with his wife (who does not know his HIV status).	Should you tell the wife that her husband is HIV positive?	First, encourage the patient to disclose his HIV status to his wife and set up an appointment for both in your office to be sure he follows through and to answer the wife's questions. If he refuses to tell his wife you must tell her, because his behavior poses a significant threat to her life. If he is using condoms, you do not have to inform her of his HIV-positive status.

HIV = human immunodeficiency virus; AIDS = acquired immune deficiency syndrome.